8545_GWV_Scherl

Holger Scherl

Evaluation of State-of-the-Art Hardware Architectures
for Fast Cone-Beam CT Reconstruction

VIEWEG+TEUBNER RESEARCH

Medizintechnik – Medizinische Bildgebung, Bildverarbeitung und bildgeführte Interventionen

Herausgegeben von Prof. Dr. Thorsten M. Buzug,
Institut für Medizintechnik, Universität zu Lübeck

Die medizinische Bildgebung erforscht, mit welchen Wechselwirkungen zwischen Energie und Gewebe räumlich aufgelöste Signale von Zellen oder Organen gewonnen werden können, die die Form oder Funktion eines Organs charakterisieren. Die Bildverarbeitung erlaubt es, die in physikalischen Messsignalen und gewonnenen Bildern enthaltene Information zu extrahieren, für den Betrachter aufzubereiten sowie automatisch zu interpretieren. Beide Gebiete stützen sich auf das Zusammenwirken der Fächer Mathematik, Physik, Informatik und Medizin und treiben als Querschnittsdisziplinen die Entwicklung der Gerätetechnologie voran.
Die Reihe Medizintechnik bietet jungen Wissenschaftlerinnen und Wissenschaftlern ein Forum, ausgezeichnete Arbeiten der Fachöffentlichkeit vorzustellen, sie steht auch Tagungsbänden offen.

Holger Scherl

Evaluation of State-of-the-Art Hardware Architectures for Fast Cone-Beam CT Reconstruction

With a foreword by Prof. Dr.-Ing. Joachim Hornegger

VIEWEG+TEUBNER RESEARCH

Bibliographic information published by the Deutsche Nationalbibliothek
The Deutsche Nationalbibliothek lists this publication in the Deutsche Nationalbibliografie;
detailed bibliographic data are available in the Internet at http://dnb.d-nb.de.

Dissertation University of Erlangen-Nuremberg, 2010

1st Edition 2011

All rights reserved
© Vieweg+Teubner Verlag | Springer Fachmedien Wiesbaden GmbH 2011

Editorial Office: Ute Wrasmann | Britta Göhrisch-Radmacher

Vieweg+Teubner Verlag is a brand of Springer Fachmedien.
Springer Fachmedien is part of Springer Science+Business Media.
www.viewegteubner.de

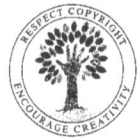
Cover design: KünkelLopka Medienentwicklung, Heidelberg
Printed on acid-free paper

ISBN 978-3-8348-1743-3

Preface by the Series Editor

The book Evaluation of State-of-the-Art Hardware Architectures for Fast Cone-Beam CT Reconstruction by Dr. Holger Scherl is the second volume of the new "Vieweg+Teubner" series of excellent theses in medical engineering. The thesis of Dr. Holger Scherl has been selected by an editorial board of highly recognized scientists working in that field.

The "Vieweg+Teubner" series aims to establish a well defined forum for monographs and proceedings on medical engineering. The series publishes works that give insights into the novel developments with emphasis on imaging, image computing and image-guided intervention.

Prospective authors may contact the series editor about future publications within the series at:

Prof. Dr. Thorsten M. Buzug
Series Editor Medical Engineering

Institute of Medical Engineering
University of Lübeck
Ratzeburger Allee 160
23562 Lübeck
Web: www.imt.uni-luebeck.de
Email: buzug@imt.uni-luebeck.de

Lübeck, 2011-04-11   Prof. Dr. Thorsten M. Buzug

Foreword by Professor Joachim Hornegger

Computed tomography is no longer limited to diagnostic imaging procedures but is nowadays routinely used in interventional radiology. The key requirement of interventional radiologists is a reconstruction time of less than 30 seconds. The usage of hardware accelerators and the development of highly optimized reconstruction algorithms is therefore not an option but mandatory from a practitioner's point of view. Especially the extension of C-arm devices with 3-D imaging capabilities has increased the demands on fast and efficient 3-D reconstruction machines. The assessment of the wide range of modern hardware accelerators for computed tomography is an emerging field. Many research teams work world wide on this problem. The large number of scientific publications on hardware accelerated 3-D reconstruction demonstrates the strong activities in this field. Most of the research is accompanied by industry that has an enormous pressure to get access to low-cost and high performance solutions.

In this book Dr. Holger Scherl considers the field of computed tomography including a review of state-of-the-art reconstruction algorithms and a concise assessment of the most recent hardware architectures. The text introduces the reader to the reconstruction problem in computed tomography and its major scientific challenges that range from computational efficiency to the fulfillment of Tuy's sufficiency condition. The assessed hardware architectures include multi- and many core systems, cell broad-band engine architecture, graphics processing units (GPUs), and field programmable gate arrays. The focus of this book is on the interplay of these recent hardware platforms and modern computed tomography reconstruction algorithms.

Dr. Scherl developed and evaluated a hard- and software framework that is unique and serves as a base for several research projects that deal with hardware accelerated reconstruction. Today the developed system is also used within product implementations in industry, and this particular transfer of the software platform from research to industry is exceptional. The pioneering work is not only appreciated by industry but also by the research community. Holger Scherl's initial publication on the GPU implementation of the reconstruction pipeline using CUDA is referenced more than 50 times.

I consider this book to be unique both in the degree of detail in the experimental evaluation and in the algorithms used for assessment. To my knowledge Holger Scherl is the first researcher considering both modern hardware architectures and most recent computed tomography algorithms.

I am pretty much convinced that the reader of this book will experience many novel aspects of computed tomography algorithms and their implementation on different hardware architectures.

Erlangen, 2011-04-04   Prof. Dr.-Ing. Joachim Hornegger

Acknowledgments

I would like to thank my advisor Prof. Dr. Joachim Hornegger (LME, University of Erlangen-Nuremberg) for introducing me to the challenging research area of medical imaging and image reconstruction in computed tomography. Thank you for your support during my time as a graduate student in your research group. I am deeply grateful for your friendly assistance and your constant encourougement to all concerns about research related issues and private matters! I also wish to thank Prof. Dr. Arndt Bode (LRR, TU Munich) for reviewing this thesis.

I wish to give very special thanks to Dr. Markus Kowarschik (Siemens Healthcare) for his guidance and motivating influence on my work. I have enjoyed our numerous and valuable scientific discussions throughout the years. He further did a great job in proofreading all parts of this thesis.

Furthermore, I would like to thank all my current and former colleagues and friends of the LME team. I would like to express my gratitude to Dr. Stefan Hoppe, Benjamin Keck (LME, University of Erlangen), Hannes Hofmann (LME, University of Erlangen) and Dr. Marcus Prümmer (LME, University of Erlangen) for the friendly and productive collaboration. Thank you very much for your cooperativeness which I have deeply appreciated!

In particular, I would like to strongly emphasize and to express my gratitude to all the students with whom I had the pleasure to collaborate over the last few years: Mario Körner, Hannes Hofmann, Mikulas Kovac, Rüdiger Bock, Sebastian Sauer, Rainer Grimmer and Gunnar Payer contributed many important pieces to my research that has finally led to the writing of this thesis.

I am further indebted to Dr. Wieland Eckert (Siemens Healthcare) for the great opportunity to contribute to the evaluation of the Cell processor. Moreover, I owe thanks to Dr. Günter Lauritsch (Siemens Healthcare) and Dr. Holger Kunze (Siemens Healthcare) for their constant willingness to discuss complex issues in the field of computed tomography. I also owe thanks to Dr. Klaus Engel for rendering the images of the reconstructed volume datasets, which are presented in the Appendix.

Finally, I would like to thank the Siemens AG for providing financial support for my research.

Last not least, I express my deep gratitude to my wife Claudia. Thanks for your patience and for your invaluable support!

Erlangen, 2010-04-26   Holger Scherl

Abstract

We present an evaluation of state-of-the-art computer hardware architectures for implementing the FDK method, which solves the three-dimensional image reconstruction task in cone-beam computed tomography (CT). The computational complexity of the FDK method prohibits its use for many clinical applications unless appropriate hardware acceleration is employed. Today's most powerful hardware architectures for high-performance computing applications are based on standard multi-core processors, off-the-shelf graphics boards, the Cell Broadband Engine Architecture (CBEA), or customized accelerator platforms (e.g., FPGA-based computer components).

For each hardware platform under consideration, we describe a thoroughly optimized implementation of the most time-consuming parts of the FDK method; the filtering step as well as the subsequent back-projection step. We further explain the required code transformations to parallelize the algorithm for the respective target architecture. We compare both the implementation complexity and the resulting performance of all architectures under consideration using the same two medical datasets which have been acquired using a standard C-arm device. Our optimized back-projection implementations achieve at least a speed-up of 6.5 (CBEA), 22.0 (GPU), and 35.8 (FPGA) compared to a standard workstation equipped with a quad-core processor. It is demonstrated that three hardware platforms (namely CBEA, GPUs, and FPGA-based architectures) enable real-time CT reconstruction and therefore support highly efficient clinical workflow.

We further describe and evaluate an optimized CBEA-based implementation of the M-line method, which is a theoretically exact and stable reconstruction algorithm. The M-line method solves the problem of cone-artifacts, which may cover small object details, thus providing excellent image quality. Its implementation, however, has an increased computational complexity as the M-line method requires additional computations for the filtering of the projection images, e.g. derivative computation and filtering along oblique lines in the projections. The execution time of filtering increases by a factor of 3.5 compared to the FDK method. Nevertheless, we are able to demonstrate on-the-fly rconstruction capability on a dual Cell Blade.

Finally, we present an efficient implementation of the computationally most demanding steps in iterative reconstruction algorithms on off-the-shelf graphics boards. Because the back-projection step can be implemented similar to the FDK method we especially consider the forward-projection step. Our implementation is based on a ray casting algorithm in order to make efficient use of the texture hardware in current graphics accelerators. Using a reasonable parameter configuration the forward-projection step requires roughly twice as much processing time as the back-projection step.

Kurzfassung

Wir präsentieren eine Evaluierung verschiedener moderner Computerarchitekturen zur Implementierung der FDK Methode, die das dreidimensionale Rekonstruktionsproblem in der Computertomographie aus Kegelstrahlprojektionen löst. Die Rechenkomplexität der FDK Methode verhindert deren Einsatz in vielen klinischen Applikationen, solange keine geeignete Hardwarebeschleunigung eingesetzt wird. Heutzutage basieren die meisten Hardwarearchitekturen, die für hochperformante Rechenanwendungen geeignet sind, auf gewöhnlichen Mehrkernprozessoren, auf der Cell Broadband Engine Architektur (CBEA), auf Standardgrafikbeschleunigerkarten oder auf maßgeschneiderten Beschleunigerarchitekturen wie beispielsweise FPGA-basierten Computerkomponenten. Wir beschreiben für jede betrachtete Hardwarearchitektur eine sorgfältig optimierte Implementierung der rechenaufwändigsten Schritte der FDK Methode: der Filterschritt sowie auch der darauffolgende Rückprojektionsschritt. Wir zeigen außerdem notwendige Codetransformationen um den Algorithmus für die einzelnen Zielarchitekturen zu parallelisieren. Wir vergleichen sowohl die Komplexität der Implementierungen als auch die erzielte Performanz aller betrachteter Architekturen anhand zweier medizinischer Datensätze, die mit einem C-Bogengerät aufgenommen wurden. Unsere optimierten Rückprojektionsimplementierungen erzielen im Vergleich zu einer Standard-Workstation mit einem Vierkernprozessor mindestens eine Beschleunigung um den Faktor 6.5 (CBEA), 22.0 (GPU) und 35.8 (FPGA). Es konnte gezeigt werden, dass drei Hardwareplattformen (CBEA, GPUs und FPGA-basierte Architekturen) eine CT-Rekonstruktion in Echtzeit ermöglichen und damit sehr effizient den klinischen Arbeitsablauf unterstützen.

Weiterhin beschreiben und evaluieren wir eine optimierte CBEA-basierte Implementierung der M-line Methode, die ein theoeretisch exaktes und stabiles Rekonstruktionsverfahren darstellt. Die M-line Methode liefert eine exzellente Bildqualität, da sie das Problem der Kegelstrahlartefakte, die kleine Objektdetails verdecken können, löst. Ihre Implementierung verlangt jedoch eine erhöhte Rechenkomplexität, weil die M-line Methode zusätzliche Berechnungen für die Filterung von Projektionsbildern erfordert, wie zum Beispiel die Berechnung von Ableitungen und die Filterung entlang schräger Linien innerhalb einer Projektion. Im Vergleich zur FDK Methode erhöht sich die Ausführungszeit der Filterung um den Faktor 3.5. Wir können dennoch auf einem dualen Cell Blade eine mit der Datenaufnahme schritthaltende Rekonstruktion erzielen.

Schließlich präsentieren wir eine effiziente Implementierung der rechenintensivsten Schritte eines iterativen Rekonstruktionsalgorithmus auf Standardgrafikbeschleunigern. Hierbei betrachten wir besonders den Vorwärtsprojektionsschritt. Die Implementierung des Rückprojektionsschrittes ist nahezu identisch mit deren Implementierung im Falle der FDK Methode. Um die Textureinheiten in aktuellen Grafikprozessoren effizient nutzen zu können, basiert unsere Implementierung auf einem sogenannten Strahlverfolgungsverfahren (ray casting). Unter Benutzung einer adäquaten Parameterkonfiguration benötigt der Vorwärtsprojektionsschritt ungefähr doppelt so viel Verarbeitungszeit wie der Rückprojektionsschritt.

Contents

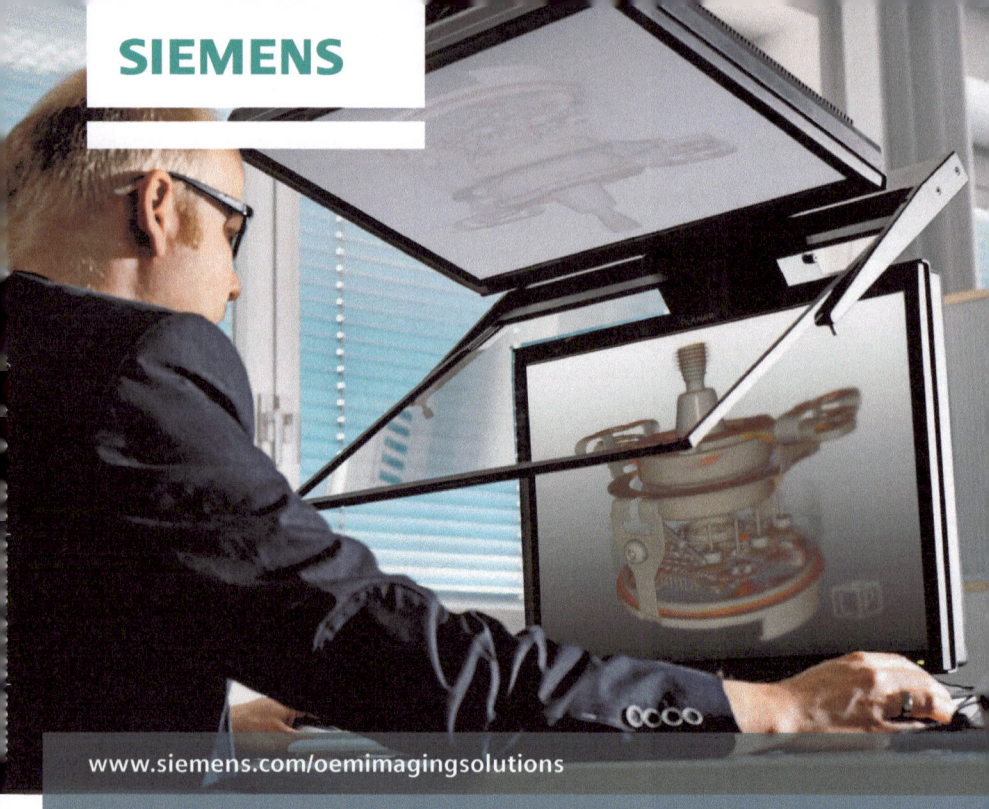

Chapter 1

Introduction

Computed tomography (CT) is a widely used imaging technique in the field of medical diagnosis and industrial non-destructive testing (NDT) applications. Using a sufficiently large series of X-ray images taken from different views around the object or patient a digital computer is used to generate slice images of the inside of the considered object or patient.

In modern CT devices three-dimensional (3-D) reconstruction techniques are employed that are able to deal with the cone-beam geometry resulting from X-ray projections that are measured with a two-dimensional detector array. This imaging approach enables the fast acquisition of the projection images and at the same time delivers high image quality. The computational complexity of the applied 3-D reconstruction methods prohibits their use in many medical applications without hardware acceleration. The use of hardware acceleration is therefore an important area of research in the field of cone-beam reconstruction. It is very important that advances in the theory of 3-D reconstruction go hand in hand with the development of suitable parallelization techniques that map them efficiently to appropriate hardware acceleration platforms.

1.1 Reconstruction Algorithms

A computationally efficient way to solve the reconstruction task is a technique which is called filtered back-projection (FBP). FBP methods achieve the reconstruction of an object by first filtering the cone-beam projections and then computing the back-projection of the filtered projections into the 3-D space.

The most successful full 3-D FBP algorithm was developed by Feldkamp, Davis, and Kress, which is commonly referred to as the FDK method [Feld 84]. The algorithm deals with a circular acquisition trajectory, where the X-ray source and the detector rotate around the center of the object to be scanned. It is equally possible to fix the X-ray source and detector while rotating the object, which is often the case in NDT applications.

The FDK method is used in most of today's cone-beam CT scanners such as C-arm devices, radiation therapy devices, dental CT devices, and in a modified way also in 3-D digital mammography devices and helical CT scanners (see Figure 1.1) as the standard image reconstruction approach.

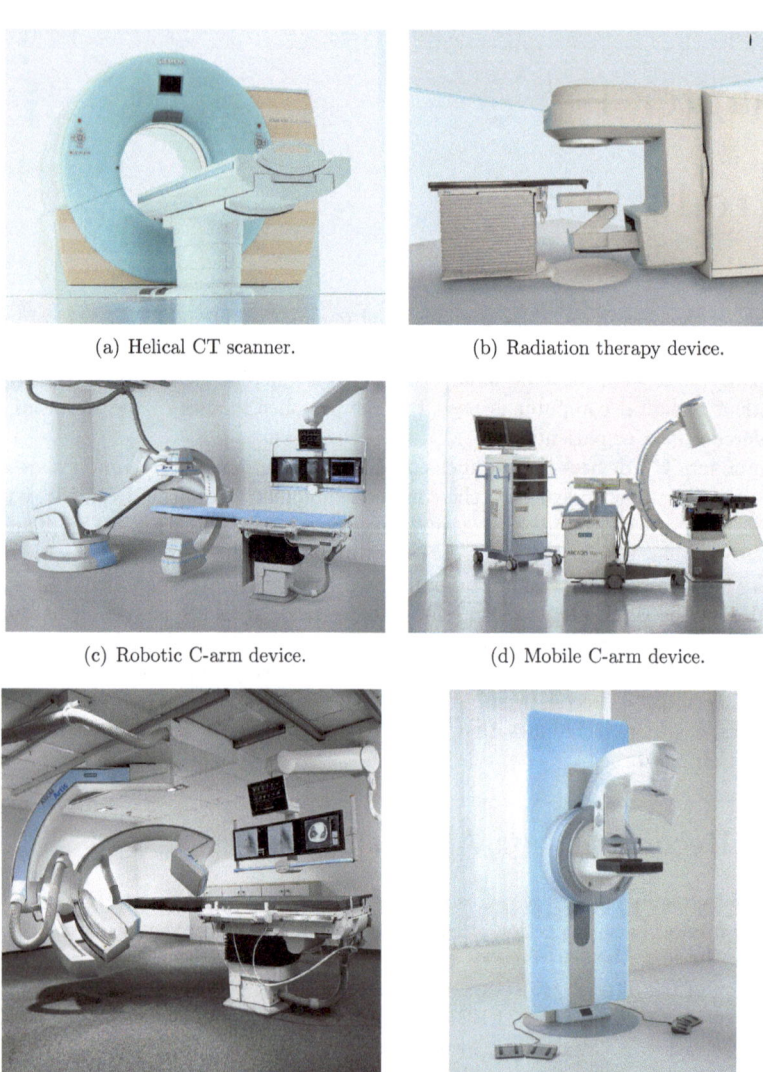

(a) Helical CT scanner.

(b) Radiation therapy device.

(c) Robotic C-arm device.

(d) Mobile C-arm device.

(e) Ceiling-mounted C-arm device.

(f) Digital mammography device (3-D breast tomosynthesis).

Figure 1.1: Several medical devices using CT imaging. By courtesy of Siemens AG.

In medical imaging a high image quality is required. Using the state-of-the-art FDK method, however, the occurring cone artifacts may cover small object details complicating their distinction. Cone artifacts manifest in the reconstruction as blurred zones at high density contrasts in the direction of the rotation axis. In medical datasets high density contrasts are located mainly at the transition between bone structures and tissue or air. The approximative nature of the Feldkamp algorithm is due to two reasons. First, the circular acquisition does not fulfill the data completeness condition necessary to compute a 3-D reconstruction using cone-beam measurements [Tuy 83], and second, the applied theory is a rather straightforward extension of the 2-D reconstruction theory to the 3-D geometry [Turb 01]. This adaption is incorrect in a strictly mathematical sense, but it still provides acceptable image quality in many medical and industrial application areas.

Recently, theoretically exact and stable[1] reconstruction algorithms have been developed providing excellent image quality without any cone artifacts and at the same time allowing an implementation in the computationally efficient FBP framework. Nevertheless, these algorithms have an increased computational complexity as they require additional computations for the filtering of the projection images, e.g. derivative computation and filtering along oblique lines in the projection. Thus, especially the filtering of projections incurs much more computations to be performed by the image reconstruction hardware. In order to apply these methods to cone-beam CT the data completeness condition must be ensured (see [Scho 01] for an overview of complete source trajectories). For example, appropriate trajectories are provided by a helical acquisition [Kats 03] or by extending the circular acquisition with an additional line [Kats 04] or arc segment [Kats 05].

The reconstruction task can also be solved in an entirely different way using iterative reconstruction methods. These methods start from an initial volume to be reconstructed. Then, a sequence of alternating forward-projections of the current reconstructed object and a corrective back-projection is performed until the reconstruction has converged to a solution that fits a certain convergence criterion. While iterative approaches are conceptually simpler than analytical approaches, they are computationally much more demanding, which has prohibited their use in most practical CT reconstruction systems up to now. However, in certain situations improved image quality can be achieved by using iterative approaches [Muel 98]. This is especially the case when a sufficiently large number of projections is not feasible or simply not desired to measure. Iterative approaches further achieve better image quality when the projections are not uniformly distributed over the scan trajectory. Statistical iterative reconstruction approaches have been used in molecular imaging scanners for a few years. In this domain it is possible to significantly improve the image quality for noisy data by incorporating physical effects of the acquisition process into the reconstruction algorithm.

---

[1] A reconstruction algorithm is theoretically exact and stable when the reconstruction is consistent, i.e., identical to the ground truth when the algorithm is applied to noise-free data with infinite spatial and temporal resolution, and when the reconstruction is stable, i.e., robust for finite resolution effects and data noise [Noo 09].

1.2 Hardware Variants

The typical clinical workflow requires high-speed reconstructions in order to enable high patient throughput or to avoid an interruption of patient treatment during interventional procedures. From the physician's perspective, it is required that the computation of the reconstructed volume from a set of acquired two-dimensional X-ray projections terminates roughly with the end of the scanning period so that no additional time delay is experienced and the volume dataset can be analyzed immediately after the scan.

The computational complexity of the algorithms mentioned in the previous section depends linearly on both the number of projection images that are acquired during the scan period as well as the number of voxels of the volume dataset to be reconstructed. In order to fulfill the physician's challenging performance requirements, it is inevitable to employ fast compute hardware. There is in fact a variety of compute hardware that can be employed to design high-speed image reconstruction systems. We are going to evaluate following hardware variants in this thesis (see also Figure 1.2):

1. The amazing progress in VLSI design[2] has led to the development of micro-processors consisting of several independent compute cores that can execute multiple application tasks in parallel. The cores belonging to one *central processing unit (CPU)* often share certain levels of the on-chip memory hierarchy (e.g., on-chip Level 2 (L2) caches). These processors are commonly referred to as *multi-core* or even as *many-core CPUs*. Current CPU manufacturers such as Intel and AMD currently provide up to eight compute cores per CPU with forecasts predicting 32 and even more parallel cores per CPU chip.

2. The *Cell Broadband Engine Architecture (CBEA)*, which was developed by IBM, Sony, and Toshiba, represents a special member of the family of multi-core CPUs. The CBEA is characterized by an architecture that covers a control core as well as eight high-performance processing cores. While the CBEA primarily targets the gaming industry, it has been demonstrated that this architecture is suitable for various numerically intensive applications in industrial and medical environments as well.

3. Standard graphics boards based on powerful *graphics processing units (GPUs)* can serve as another hardware alternative for high-performance computing applications. Current GPUs offer massively parallel processing capability that can particularly handle the computational complexity of three-dimensional cone-beam reconstruction. Nvidia has recently developed the fundamentally new easy-to-use computing paradigm *CUDA (Compute Unified Device Architecture)* for solving complex computational problems on the GPU. CUDA offers a unified hardware and software solution for parallel computing on CUDA-capable Nvidia GPUs, supporting the standard C programming language together with high-performance computing numerical libraries[3]. This enables programmers

---

[2] Very-large-scale integration (VLSI) is the process of creating integrated circuits by combining thousands of transistor-based circuits into a single chip.

[3] http://developer.nvidia.com/object/cuda.html

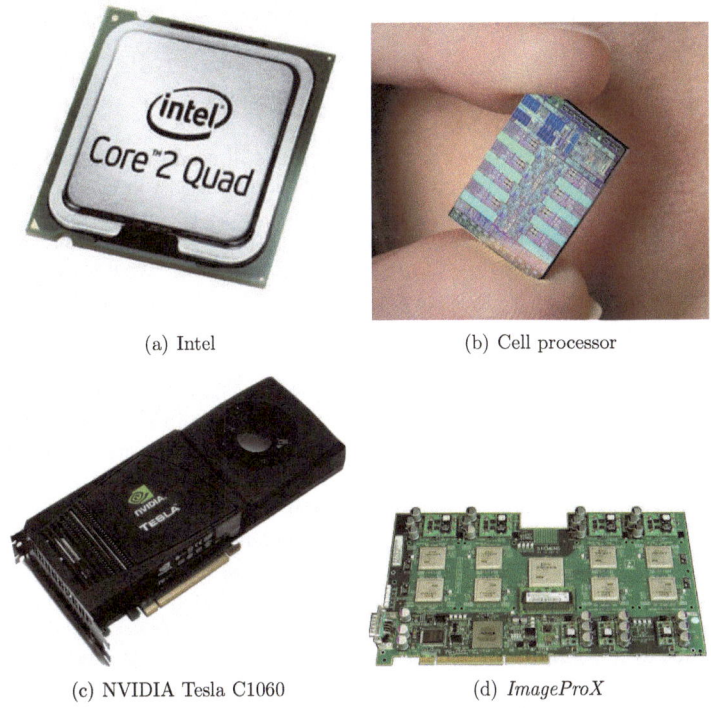

(a) Intel   (b) Cell processor

(c) NVIDIA Tesla C1060   (d) *ImageProX*

Figure   1.2:   Considered   hardware   variants.   Image   (a)   is   taken
from   http://www.intel.com/pressroom/kits/quadcore/index.htm,   Image   (b)   is
taken from http://en.wikipedia.org/wiki/File:Cell-Processor.jpg, and Image (d) is
by courtesy of Siemens AG.

that are not specialists in computer graphics to benefit from the processing
power of graphics cards. The implementation of the reconstruction task can
now be accomplished without knowing how to (ab)use the existing application
programming interfaces for general-purpose computing; e.g., OpenGL, DirectX,
or the Brook language.

4. Reconfigurable microchips represent another architecture alternative for accel-
   erating numerically intensive algorithms. *FPGAs (field-programmable gate ar-*
   rays) and *CPLDs (complex programmable logic devices)* are the most promi-
   nent representatives of reconfigurable circuits [Meye 08]. In general, FPGAs
   are characterized by a larger number of arithmetic units than CPLDs. Several
   independent vendors offer FPGA-based accelerator cards for use in general-
   purpose computer environments, along with appropriate development kits for
   software and firmware. Today, many CT devices employ FPGA hardware for

image reconstruction that has been developed by the manufacturer of the CT system itself in order to precisely meet the manufacturer's requirements.

1.3   Related Work

Published results using PC-based implementations still need more than several minutes for the reconstruction at high spatial resolution such as volumes of 512^3 voxels or even more [Wies 00, Yu 01, Kach 06]. Therefore, many specialized hardware platforms have been designed in the past to reconstruct volumes from cone-beam projections, ranging from dedicated hardware solutions like FPGAs [Trep 02, Godd 02, Heig 07] and "digital signal processors" (DSPs) [Neri 07, Lian 10] to clusters of workstations [Reim 96, Laur 98].

Recently, a flat-panel cone-beam back-projection was published using one of the two Cell processors of a dual Cell Blade [Kach 07]. The results are comparable to the performance of our Cell-based back-projection module in this thesis. The same implementation approach was used in [Yan 08, Xu 07] demonstrating a graphics-based implementation using OpenGL.

The most time-consuming operation in the inner loop of reconstruction is the ratio computation due to the non-linear perspective projection model. Our approach avoids image rectification as suggested by [Ridd 06] and used by [Kach 07, Yan 08, Xu 07] that leads to the elimination of the homogeneous division, but introduces an additional low-pass filtering operation on the projection.

In order to implement the back-projection on GPUs, OpenGL and shading languages are still used in many publications [Muel 07, Chur 07]. In comparison to the traditional graphics-based implementation methods, our CUDA-based implementation of cone-beam reconstruction has even a slightly improved reconstruction speed.

In [Hill 09] an interesting GPU-based reconstruction approach is demonstrated which does a high-speed reconstruction of an arbitrary volume slice on-demand when it is requested by the visualization software.

Only few publications, however, address all time-consuming reconstruction tasks, filtering and back-projection, in a single publication. Moreover, a direct comparison of these results is not always possible in an objective manner since different algorithms, datasets and acquisition geometries were used.

1.4   Scope and Main Contribution of this Thesis

This thesis presents a detailed overview of the aforementioned hardware platforms and their application to the three-dimensional image reconstruction task in CT.

In the first part of this thesis, we develop and evaluate an implementation approach for the most commonly used reconstruction algorithm in practical cone-beam CT scanners; the FDK method. We outline the challenges to implement this algorithm for real CT systems that usually deviate slightly from the ideal Feldkamp geometry. In this regard the main contribution of this thesis, however, can be classified as a thorough optimization and evaluation of computational performance using different hardware platforms. Several parallel implementations are developed – each of them is specially suited for one of the mentioned acceleration devices. Our optimized implementation of the FDK method has been presented at the SPIE Medical Imaging Conference 2007 [Sche 07c] for the CBEA and for graphics accelerators at the IEEE Nuclear Science Symposium and Medical Imaging Conference 2007 [Sche 07b]. These implementations enable a novel reconstruction mode where an FDK reconstruction is computed on-the-fly at the same time the data is acquired by the C-arm device. The reconstructed volume can thus be shown to the physician in real time immediately after the last projection image has been acquired.

During our evaluations we use the same two medical datasets, which were acquired using a standard C-arm device, on each of the considered hardware platforms. Therefore, we are able to present a fair comparison of the currently most promising hardware variants in the context of cone-beam reconstruction. This is a novel practice since we use the same implementation approach of the FDK method – suitable for practical cone-beam CT scanners – and the same datasets for the evaluation of several state-of-the-art hardware architectures. This comparative study has been submitted to the Journal of Medical Physics.

We further present both the design and the implementation of a software architecture that is used by all of our optimized implementations. Software engineering techniques play an important role in the overall design and can improve the efficiency, flexibility, and portability of the whole reconstruction system. We show how this design can act as a hardware abstraction layer on top of different acceleration architectures. The design and implementation of our software architecture has been presented at the International Conference on Software Engineering 2008 [Sche 08].

Since the FDK method is of an approximative nature, its reconstruction results suffer from severe artifacts in certain situations. In the second part of this thesis we select two alternative approaches to cone-beam reconstruction, which are able to deliver significantly improved image quality when compared to the results of the FDK method.

We show for the first time a highly optimized implementation of a theoretically exact and stable FBP algorithm. We select the M-line method, which is well suited for the non-ideal acquisitions in practical cone-beam CT scanners, and at the same time totally resolves the problem of cone artifacts in FDK reconstructions. We further demonstrate on-the-fly reconstruction on a dual Cell Blade using our optimized CBEA-based implementation. The performance-optimized version of the M-line method has been presented at the International Meeting on Fully Three-Dimensional Image Reconstruction in Radiology and Nuclear Medicine 2007 [Sche 07a].

Additionally, we present an iterative reconstruction approach with a strong focus on the CUDA-based optimization of its most time-consuming processing steps; the forward-projection and the back-projection. Iterative approaches can be used when analytic algorithms such as the FDK method and the M-line method do not achieve good image quality. For example this is the case when a sufficiently large number of projections is not feasible or simply not desired to measure. Iterative approaches have also the opportunity to achieve better image quality when the projections are not uniformly distributed over the scan trajectory. Our optimized CUDA-based implementation of the forward- and back-projection module has been presented at the International Workshop on New Frontiers in High-performance and Hardware-aware

Computing 2008 [Wein 08] and at the IEEE Nuclear Science Symposium and Medical Imaging Conference 2009 [Keck 09a]. Furthermore, our optimized implementations of both the forward- and the back-projection are used in an ongoing research project at the University of Erlangen-Nuremberg, Chair of Computer Science 5 (Pattern Recognition) [Keck 09b].

1.5   Outline

The structure of this thesis is as follows. Chapter 2 describes several reconstruction methods for computing a volumetric representation of a scanned object from a set of two-dimensional X-ray projection images. In particular we present the approximate FDK method (Section 2.2), the theoretically exact and stable M-line method applied to a short-scan circle-plus-arc acquisition (Section 2.3.1) and the simultaneous algebraic reconstruction technique as a representative of the iterative approaches (Section 2.3.2).

Chapter 3 contains an overview of the underlying software layer that we have developed in order to facilitate the integration of hardware accelerators into our image reconstruction software infrastructure.

The architectures of the considered hardware variants and efficient implementations of the FDK reconstruction method on these hardware platforms are presented in Chapters 5 to 7. Each Chapter addresses a single hardware architecture.

In Chapter 4, we discuss our CBEA-based implementation and present corresponding performance results. Chapter 5 then focuses on multi-core CPUs and again summarizes our results. In Chapter 6, we outline CUDA-based implementations on Nvidia graphics cards. Chapter 7 contains a description of a highly efficient implementation using the FPGA-based hardware accelerator platform *ImageProX*, which was developed by Siemens Healthcare.

In the following chapter (Chapter 8) we focus on two alternative reconstruction algorithms. In particular we present a highly optimized CBEA-based implementation of the M-line method (Section 8.1) and a CUDA-accelerated version of the most computationally demanding processing steps of an iterative method (Section 8.2).

Finally, in Chapter 9, we compare our results, draw our final conclusions, and discuss possible future directions of research in the field of hardware-accelerated cone-beam CT reconstruction.

Chapter 2

Algorithms for Cone-Beam Image Reconstruction

There exist several reconstruction methods for computing a volumetric representation of a scanned object from a set of two-dimensional X-ray projection images. However, the most commonly applied method in practical cone-beam CT systems is the approximate FDK method. After we give some prerequisites that are necessary to understand the following descriptions, we present in Section 2.2 the FDK method, discuss possible implementation strategies (Section 2.2.2) that can be applied to practical cone-beam systems and analyze the time complexity of the involved algorithmic steps (Section 2.2.3).

Although many CT systems use the FDK method to solve the 3-D image reconstruction task, it is not without its short-comings. Therefore, we describe in Section 2.3 two alternative approaches: the theoretically exact and stable M-line method applied to a short-scan circle-plus-arc acquisition (Section 2.3.1) and the simultaneous algebraic reconstruction technique as a representative of the iterative approaches (Section 2.3.2). The M-line method totally resolves the problem of cone artifacts, which result from the approximative nature of the FDK method. Iterative approaches can be used when analytic algorithms such as the FDK method and the M-line method do not achieve good image quality. For example this is the case when a sufficiently large number of projections is not feasible or simply not desired to measure. Iterative approaches also have the opportunity to achieve better image quality when the projections are not uniformly distributed over the scan trajectory.

2.1 Prerequisites

The task in 3-D image reconstruction is to recover the function of X-ray attenuation coefficients $f(\underline{x})$ of an object under examination, provided a set of line integrals

$$g(\lambda, \underline{\theta}) = \int_0^\infty f(\underline{a}(\lambda) + t\underline{\theta})dt. \qquad (2.1)$$

Here, the 3-D curve $\underline{a}(\lambda)$ describes the corresponding position of the X-ray source with λ varying over a finite interval of $\mathbb{R}$, and the unit vector $\underline{\theta}$ represents the direction of the respective ray.

If we assume a flat-panel detector located at a distance D from the current source position, each detector value at coordinates $(u, v)^T$ refers to an integral along a straight line with direction

$$\underline{\theta}(u, v) = \left(u\underline{e}_u + v\underline{e}_v - D\underline{e}_w \right) \big/ \sqrt{u^2 + v^2 + D^2} \,. \tag{2.2}$$

Here, the detector coordinates are identified by two orthogonal unit vectors $\underline{e}_u$ and $\underline{e}_v$, and the origin $(0, 0)^T$ of the detector coordinate system (DCS) is the orthogonal projection of $\underline{a}(\lambda)$ onto the detector. The unit vector $\underline{e}_w = \underline{e}_u \times \underline{e}_v$ points from the origin of the DCS towards the source position. The ray that hits the detector at the origin of the detector coordinate system is commonly referred to as *principal ray*, while the respective intersection point is usually referred to as *principal point*. The set of rays corresponding to a certain source position $\underline{a}(\lambda)$ and a certain flat-panel detector position thus geometrically forms a cone-beam. Throughout this thesis we refer to the resulting 2-D X-ray images as cone-beam projections. This scan geometry is illustrated in Figure 2.1.

2.2 The Feldkamp Algorithm

In 1984, Feldkamp, Davis, and Kress published an algorithm for circular cone-beam tomography, which is still widely used in state-of-the-art cone-beam scanning devices; e.g., C-arm CT. This algorithm is usually referred to as *Feldkamp method* or as *FDK method* [Feld 84]. It represents an analytical 3-D reconstruction method resulting in a filtered back-projection scheme. It can be understood as an extension of exact 2-D reconstruction algorithms for fan-beam projections [Kak 01] to the 3-D case by properly adapting the weighting factors.

The Feldkamp algorithm is based upon a circular trajectory, as is shown in Figure 2.1. The X-ray source rotates along an ideal circle of radius R with center point O in the midplane about the axis of rotation that is defined by the point O and the direction $\underline{e}_z$. Each point $\underline{a}(\lambda)$ on the source trajectory with λ representing the rotation angle of the source-detector assembly expressed in radians is thus given by the vector

$$\underline{a}(\lambda) = (R\cos\lambda, R\sin\lambda, 0)^T \quad \text{for} \quad \lambda \in [0, 2\pi[\,, \tag{2.3}$$

where the coordinates on the right-hand side refer to the fixed right-handed world coordinate system defined by its origin O and the unit vectors $\underline{e}_x$, $\underline{e}_y$, and $\underline{e}_z$. Then, the aforementioned unit vectors $\underline{e}_u$, $\underline{e}_v$ and $\underline{e}_w$ are given as the rotated coordinate axes

$$\underline{e}_u(\lambda) \;=\; (-\sin\lambda, \cos\lambda, 0)^T\,, \tag{2.4}$$

$$\underline{e}_v \;=\; (0, 0, 1)^T\,, \tag{2.5}$$

$$\underline{e}_w(\lambda) \;=\; (\cos\lambda, \sin\lambda, 0)^T = \underline{e}_u(\lambda) \times \underline{e}_v\,, \tag{2.6}$$

where the coordinates on the right-hand sides again refer to the fixed world coordinate system. As is illustrated in Figure 2.1, these axes are obtained from the x-, y- and

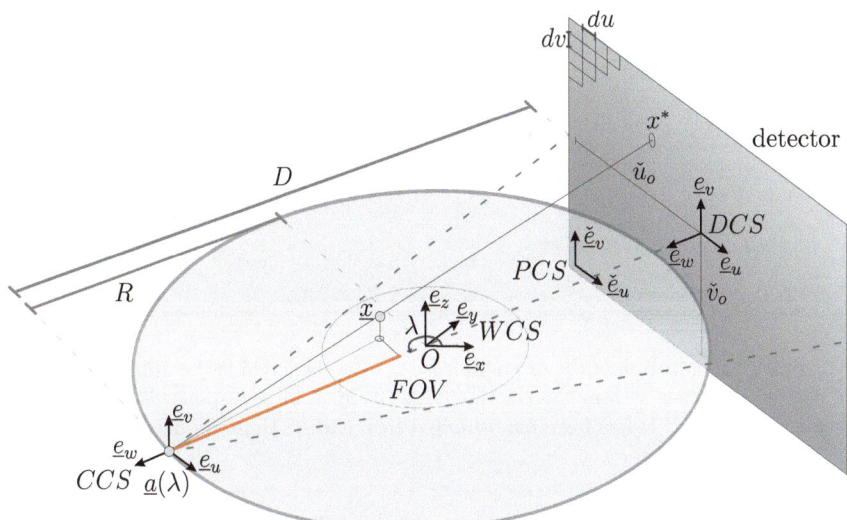

Figure 2.1: Ideal Feldkamp geometry. The X-ray source rotates along an ideal circle of radius R with center point O in the midplane about the axis of rotation that is defined by the point O and the direction $\underline{e}_z$. The rotation direction is given by the angle λ in counterclockwise direction. D is the orthogonal distance between $\underline{a}(\lambda)$ and the corresponding detector plane. Four different coordinate systems are shown: the world coordinate system (WCS), the camera coordinate system (CCS), the detector coordinate system (DCS), and the pixel coordinate system (PCS). The voxel coordinate system (VCS) is not shown in this figure. The cylindrical field-of-view (FOV) is indicated by the inner circle. Only points inside the FOV can be reconstructed.

z-axes by a rotation of angle $\pi/2 + \lambda$ about the z-axis in counter-clockwise direction and then flipping the direction of $\underline{e}_w(\lambda)$.

Throughout this thesis we use the notation " ˇ " to denote quantities that refer to coordinates of the pixel coordinate system (PCS) or the voxel coordinate system (VCS).

2.2.1 Algorithmic Steps

In order to approximately reconstruct a value $f(\underline{x})$ at any position $\underline{x} = (x, y, z)$ within the support of the object density function f using the Feldkamp algorithm, the following algorithmic steps must be applied successively[1].

---

[1] Note that the Feldkamp algorithm is only an approximate method for 3-D reconstruction. This results from the fact that a circular scan trajectory necessarily leads to an incomplete sampling of the Radon space, see [Feld 84].

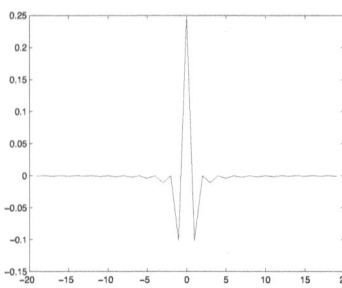 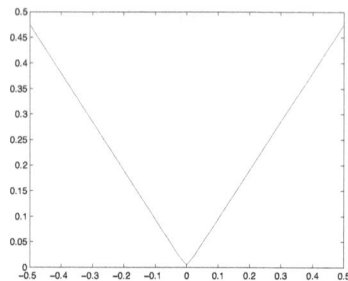

Figure 2.2: Illustration of the ramp filter h_{ramp}. On the left side the impulse response of the ramp filter is shown. On the right side the ideal filter response is shown in the frequency domain. It has been band-limited to $1/(2\,du)$. Here, du denotes the width of a pixel in direction $\underline{e}_u$.

Step 1 – Filtering.   Each projection $g(\lambda, \underline{\theta}(u, v))$ is transformed into a filtered projection $g^F(\lambda, u, v)$ according to the following steps F1 and F2:

F1 – Cosine Weighting.   Weight the data according to

$$g_1(\lambda, u, v) = \frac{D}{\sqrt{u^2 + v^2 + D^2}}\, g(\lambda, \underline{\theta}(u, v))\,, \tag{2.7}$$

where the factor $D/\sqrt{u^2 + v^2 + D^2}$ represents the cosine of the angle between the principle ray of the cone-beam hitting the detector at the origin of the DCS and the ray hitting the detector at position $(u, v)^T$, see again Figure 2.1.

F2 – Ramp Filtering.   Ramp-filter the projection images row-wise (i.e., with respect to u) by computing

$$g^F(\lambda, u, v) = g_1(\lambda, u, v) * h_{ramp}(u)\,, \tag{2.8}$$

where h_{ramp} denotes the ideal ramp filter (see Figure 2.2) and "$*$" denotes the convolution operator. This step corresponds to a 1-D convolution along lines on the detector that are parallel to $\underline{e}_u(\lambda)$.

Step 2 – Back-Projection.   Back-project the filtered projection $g^F(\lambda, u, v)$ into the image space to obtain an approximation $\hat{f}$ of f at each point $\underline{x}$ according to

$$\hat{f}(\underline{x}) = \frac{1}{2} \int_0^{2\pi} \mu(\lambda, \underline{x}) g^F(\lambda, u(\lambda, \underline{x}), v(\lambda, \underline{x})) d\lambda\,, \tag{2.9}$$

where u and v are the respective detector coordinates given by

$$u(\lambda, \underline{x}) = -D \frac{\langle (\underline{x} - \underline{a}(\lambda)), \underline{e}_u \rangle}{\langle (\underline{x} - \underline{a}(\lambda)), \underline{e}_w \rangle}\,, \tag{2.10}$$

$$v(\lambda, \underline{x}) = -D \frac{\langle (\underline{x} - \underline{a}(\lambda)), \underline{e}_v \rangle}{\langle (\underline{x} - \underline{a}(\lambda)), \underline{e}_w \rangle}\,, \tag{2.11}$$

and $\mu(\lambda, \underline{x})$ is a point-dependent distance weight according to

$$\mu(\lambda, \underline{x}) = \frac{R^2}{\langle (\underline{x} - \underline{a}(\lambda)), \underline{e}_w \rangle^2} . \tag{2.12}$$

Here, $\langle ., . \rangle$ denotes the inner product. For a detailed derivation, we refer to [Kak 01].

For short-scan acquisitions the back-projection interval has to be restricted to the covered angular range of the scan, and before the computation of (F1) an additional data redundancy weighting step, which is commonly referred to as (generalized) Parker weighting [Silv 00, Park 82] has to be applied.

In order to assess the performance using the acceleration architectures under consideration, we restrict our evaluation to the most compute-intensive algorithmic tasks; the ramp filtering step (F2) as well as the back-projection step (Step 2).

2.2.2 Implementation Strategies

2.2.2.1 Ramp Filtering

The FDK reconstruction approach requires to filter the rows of the projections using a high-pass filter in the direction of $\underline{e}_u$. An ideal acquisition would ensure that the vector $\underline{e}_u$ and thus the detector rows be parallel to the plane of the source trajectory. In practical cone-beam CT systems such as C-arm scanners this assumption may be violated due to deviations caused by mechanical inaccuracies during the acquisition process. However, we perform the ramp filtering step in the direction of the detector rows, regardless of any reconstruction inaccuracies introduced by this assumption of an ideal scan geometry[2].

Various filter kernels are used in practice; e.g. combinations of ramp filters and smoothing filters. Due to the typical filter mask sizes of 60 non-zero elements and more, convolutions are practically computed in the Fourier domain due to the reduced computational complexity. For example, considering the number of required floating-point operations for convolving a single image row with 1024 pixels the break-even point is already reached when filter mask sizes are larger than 17 pixels (see Section 2.2.3 for further details).

As is explained in detail in [Kak 01], this convolution algorithm requires the computation of the discrete Fourier transform (DFT) of each input signal (projection row) as well as the DFT of the spatial filter kernel. The actual convolution of any two vectors in Fourier space is then performed by component-wise multiplication of their Fourier components. Then, the inverse DFT (IDFT) of this product is computed in order to transform the filtered projection rows back into the spatial domain. The input vectors and the filter kernels are zero-padded up to a suitable power of two in order to avoid aliasing effects that may severely spoil the results [Gonz 08]. Throughout this thesis we denote by convolution length the zero-padded size of the input vector or filter kernel.

---

[2] In a non-ideal scan geometry it is possible that the detector rows and thus the vector $\underline{e}_u$ are slightly tilted with respect to an ideal Feldkamp-like acquisition. In such a situation the vector $\underline{e}_u$ and the geometrical parameters of the X-ray camera and the detector can be extracted from the corresponding projection matrix (see Appendix A), which is usually determined by calibration. See e.g. [Wies 00] for more details.

On the considered hardware platforms, computationally efficient FFT cores are available for the calculation of complex fast Fourier transforms (FFT). Since it is possible to compute the Fourier-based convolution for two (real-valued) input vectors simultaneously using complex FFTs, we always convolve two adjacent image rows of a projection with the given filter kernel simultaneously. One image row defines the real input while the second one refers to the imaginary input. All of our optimized implementations compute the convolution by a complex 1-D FFT followed by the point-wise multiplication of the DFT of the filter kernel and the computation of the inverse FFT (IFFT) of the respective point-wise product.

2.2.2.2   Back-Projection

Back-projection can either be implemented using a voxel- or a ray-driven volume update strategy.

In the ray-driven approach it is required to follow the rays defined by the pixels in the projection image to the source position through the volume. Each affected volume voxel gets an appropriate weighted increment depending on how much the current ray affects the respective voxel. This approach, however, is hard to parallelize for the considered hardware platforms. Each time a voxel is hit by a ray and thus gets updated, it must be ensured that no other ray does an update of that voxel at the same time. Otherwise wrong voxel accumulation may occur due to race conditions during voxel read/write accesses. Moreover, ray-based back-projection approaches tend to introduce high-frequency artifacts that manifest as Moire patterns in the final reconstruction result [De M 02, De M 04].

For these reasons, we decided to implement the voxel-driven back-projection scheme on the considered acceleration hardware. Each voxel can be updated independently by calculating the detector position where the ray emanating from the source and passing the considered voxel center hits the projection image. This results in an embarrassingly parallel problem, because projection values are accessed read-only, and all voxel accesses for the same projection are independent of each other.

Because of deviations due to mechanical inaccuracies of real cone-beam CT systems such as mobile and stationary mounted C-arm scanners, the back-projection is commonly not computed using Equations (2.9), (2.10), and (2.11) directly. Instead, the mapping between voxels of the volume and projection image positions can be described by introducing homogeneous coordinates and a corresponding 3×4 projection matrix $\mathbf{P}(\lambda)$ for each X-ray source position $\underline{a}(\lambda)$ at rotation angle λ along the trajectory [Hart 03]. The projection matrices are commonly estimated during a calibration step that must be accomplished only when the cone-beam CT scanner is installed or maintained. See for example Wiesent et al. [Wies 00] for more details about the calibration of cone-beam CT systems.

In an ideal geometry as described in Section 2.2, the projection matrices operating on points given in world coordinates can be calculated analytically from Equations (2.10) and (2.11):

$$\tilde{\mathbf{P}}(\lambda) = \begin{bmatrix} -D\sin\lambda & D\cos\lambda & 0 & 0 \\ 0 & 0 & D & 0 \\ -\cos\lambda & -\sin\lambda & 0 & R \end{bmatrix}. \tag{2.13}$$

In order to express the resulting detector coordinates with respect to the PCS, the necessary transformations can be applied by multiplying a 3×3 matrix $\tilde{\mathbf{K}}(\lambda)$ to the projection matrix of Equation (2.13) from the left[3]:

$$\mathbf{P}(\lambda) = \tilde{\mathbf{K}}(\lambda)\tilde{\mathbf{P}}(\lambda) = \begin{bmatrix} \frac{1}{du} & 0 & \check{u}_o \\ 0 & \frac{1}{dv} & \check{v}_o \\ 0 & 0 & 1 \end{bmatrix} \tilde{\mathbf{P}}(\lambda). \tag{2.14}$$

Here, du and dv denote the pixel width in u-direction and v-direction of the detector, respectively. See Figure 2.1 for a clarification of the symbols used in Equations (2.13) and (2.14). This step transforms world coordinates into pixel coordinates and translates any possible offset of the principal point. See Appendix A for further details.

Likewise the projection matrix can be modified by multiplying a 4×4-matrix from the right in order to include the necessary transformations from voxel coordinates to world coordinates. This transform comprises the necessary scaling and translation of the voxel coordinates to a representation in the world coordinate system:

$$\mathbf{T}(\lambda) = \begin{bmatrix} dx & 0 & 0 & t_x \\ 0 & dy & 0 & t_y \\ 0 & 0 & dz & t_z \\ 0 & 0 & 0 & 1 \end{bmatrix}. \tag{2.15}$$

Here, dx, dy, and dz denote the voxel widths in x-, y-, and z-direction of the world coordinate system, respectively, while t_x, t_y, and t_z represent the translation of the voxel coordinate system relative to the world coordinate system in units of world coordinates.

The final projection matrix operating on points given in voxel coordinates in an ideal Feldkamp-like acquisition is then given as

$$\check{\mathbf{P}}(\lambda) = \mathbf{P}(\lambda)\mathbf{T}(\lambda). \tag{2.16}$$

Back-projection may now be computed by calculating a matrix-vector product for each voxel and each projection in order to determine the corresponding homogeneous representation of the projection value, followed by the homogeneous division to reveal the actual detector position (see Algorithm 1)[4]. The intermediate results $\check{u}$ and $\check{v}$ represent detector positions given as column index and row index, respectively, as non-integer numbers. The computation of the actual voxel increment is hidden behind the function "fetch" that may be based on nearest neighbor or bilinear interpolation of the filtered projection values, for example.

---

[3]Note that in an ideal setting $\tilde{\mathbf{K}}(\lambda)$ covers a scaling operation and a translation operation only.

[4]Any matrix entry is referenced by its row index and its column index. $\mathbf{P}[i,j]$ thus refers to the entry in the ith row and the jth column. Throughout this thesis, arrays are assumed to be 0-based. Consequently, $\mathbf{P}[0,0]$ refers to the upper left entry of matrix $\mathbf{P}$.

Algorithm 1: Voxel-driven back-projection.

Input: N_p filtered projection images I_i, $0 \leq i < N_p$

Input: N_p projection matrices $\check{\mathbf{P}}_i$, $0 \leq i < N_p$

Data: volume $\mathbf{V}$ consisting of $N_x \times N_y \times N_z$ voxels

1 **for** $(i = 0; i < N_p; i = i + 1)$ **do**

2   **for** $(\check{z} = 0; \check{z} < N_z; \check{z} = \check{z} + 1)$ **do**

3   **for** $(\check{y} = 0; \check{y} < N_y; \check{y} = \check{y} + 1)$ **do**

4   **for** $(\check{x} = 0; \check{x} < N_x; \check{x} = \check{x} + 1)$ **do**

         // Compute homogeneous image coordinates

5          $r = \check{\mathbf{P}}_i[0,0] \cdot \check{x} + \check{\mathbf{P}}_i[0,1] \cdot \check{y} + \check{\mathbf{P}}_i[0,2] \cdot \check{z} + \check{\mathbf{P}}_i[0,3]$;

6          $s = \check{\mathbf{P}}_i[1,0] \cdot \check{x} + \check{\mathbf{P}}_i[1,1] \cdot \check{y} + \check{\mathbf{P}}_i[1,2] \cdot \check{z} + \check{\mathbf{P}}_i[1,3]$;

7          $t = \check{\mathbf{P}}_i[2,0] \cdot \check{x} + \check{\mathbf{P}}_i[2,1] \cdot \check{y} + \check{\mathbf{P}}_i[2,2] \cdot \check{z} + \check{\mathbf{P}}_i[2,3]$;

8          $t_{inv} = 1/t$;

9          $\check{u} = r \cdot t_{inv}$;   // Dehomogenize

10         $\check{v} = s \cdot t_{inv}$;   // Dehomogenize

11         $\mu = t_{inv} \cdot t_{inv}$;   // Distance weight

12         $\mathbf{V}[\check{x}, \check{y}, \check{z}] = \mathbf{V}[\check{x}, \check{y}, \check{z}] + \mu \cdot \text{fetch}(I_i, \check{u}, \check{v})$;   // Accumulate

13   **end**

14   **end**

15   **end**

16 **end**

For neighboring voxels, it is sufficient to increment the homogeneous detector coordinates by the appropriate column of $\check{\mathbf{P}}(\lambda)$ [Wies 00]. Algorithm 2 shows the pseudo-code for the computationally optimized version (incremental version) of the back-projection step. First, we calculate in each loop the base increment for the homogeneous detector coordinates. Then, in each loop we multiply the actual voxel index with the respective voxel increments before adding them to the base increments of the current loop. This approach requires an additional floating-point multiplication for each voxel to compute the homogeneous detector coordinates. We avoid to simply increment the actual computed homogeneous detector coordinates, which would save the additional floating-point operation but introduces numerical problems. The hardware variants, which we consider throughout this thesis, provide a special multiply-add floating-point operation such that both approaches require only a single instruction.

The homogeneous divide operation in Algorithm 2 cannot be avoided for voxel position increments parallel to the z-axis of the VCS because, in practical cone-beam CT systems, the projection planes are slightly tilted with respect to the z-axis due mechanical inaccuracies. We intentionally avoided the use of a detector rebinning technique that virtually aligns the detector to one of the volume axis because it impairs the resulting image quality and requires additional computations for the initial rebinning step [Ridd 06].

Note that, in Algorithm 1 and Algorithm 2, the voxel-specific distance weight $\mu = \mu(\lambda, \underline{x})$ is determined by exploiting a computational trick. Since each projection

---

Algorithm 2: Incremental version of voxel-driven back-projection.

Input: N_p filtered projection images I_i, $0 \leq i < N_p$
Input: N_p projection matrices $\check{\mathbf{P}}_i$, $0 \leq i < N_p$
Data: volume $\mathbf{V}$ consisting of $N_x \times N_y \times N_z$ voxels

```
 1 for (i = 0; i < Np; i = i + 1) do
 2     for (ž = 0; ž < Nz; ž = ž + 1) do
            // Compute z-increments
 3         rz = P̌i[0,2] · ž + P̌i[0,3];
 4         sz = P̌i[1,2] · ž + P̌i[1,3];
 5         tz = P̌i[2,2] · ž + P̌i[2,3];
 6         for ( y̌ = 0; y̌ < Ny; y̌ = y̌ + 1) do
                // Compute y-increments
 7             ry = P̌i[0,1] · y̌ + rz;
 8             sy = P̌i[1,1] · y̌ + sz;
 9             ty = P̌i[2,1] · y̌ + tz;
10             for x̌ = 0; x̌ < Nx; x̌ = x̌ + 1) do
                    // Compute homogeneous image coordinates
11                 r = P̌i[0,0] · x̌ + ry;
12                 s = P̌i[1,0] · x̌ + sy;
13                 t = P̌i[2,0] · x̌ + ty;
14                 tinv = 1/t;
15                 ǔ = r · tinv;                      // Dehomogenize
16                 v̌ = s · tinv;                      // Dehomogenize
17                 μ = tinv · tinv;                   // Distance weight
18                 V[x̌, y̌, ž] = V[x̌, y̌, ž] + μ · fetch(Ii, ǔ, v̌);   // Accumulate
19             end
20         end
21     end
22 end
```

---

matrix $\mathbf{P}(\lambda)$ is only defined up to a scale factor, we normalize $\mathbf{P}(\lambda)$ such that $\mathbf{P}(\lambda)[2,3] = 1$. In this case, it follows from Equations (2.12) and (2.14) that

$$\mu(\lambda, \underline{x}) = \frac{R^2}{\langle(\underline{x} - \underline{a}(\lambda)), \underline{e}_w\rangle^2} = \frac{1}{t^2}. \tag{2.17}$$

Consequently, only one additional multiply operation is necessary to compute the distance weight itself (i.e., $t^{-1} \cdot t^{-1}$) and another one to compute the weighted voxel increment $\mu \cdot \text{fetch}(I_i, \check{u}, \check{v})$ afterwards.

2.2.3 Complexity Analysis

In the last section we presented implementation approaches for the two most time-consuming processing steps of filtered back-projection algorithms; the filtering step as well as the subsequent back-projection step. In this section we will analyze their time complexity.

2.2.3.1   Filtering

As mentioned in Section 2.2.2.1 the filtering step can be implemented in the spatial or in the frequency domain. In the following we estimate the number of required floating-point operations required to implement each variant.

In the spatial domain the 1-D discrete convolution of the image rows of g with a filter kernel given as a 1-D mask h and consisting of $N_M = 2m + 1$ elements (cf. Equation 2.8) can be computed by

$$g(\check{u}, \check{v}) = \sum_{k=-m}^{m} h(k) g(\check{u} - k, \check{v}) \,. \tag{2.18}$$

The convolution for an image pixel requires one multiplication and one addition for each mask element, which results in

$$N_{spatial} = 2 N_M N_u N_v N_p \tag{2.19}$$

floating-point operations for N_p projection images consisting of N_v rows and N_u columns. With $N = N_u = N_v = N_p$ the discrete 1-D convolution of the projection image rows in the spatial domain has a time complexity of $\mathcal{O}(N^3)$ for filter kernels with fixed impulse.

In the following we analyze the number of required floating-point operations when computing the 1-D convolution in the frequency domain. In order to transform an image row into the frequency domain and back to the spatial domain two FFTs have to be computed. The classic "radix-2" algorithm presented by Cooley and Tukey [Cool 65] requires a number of floating-point operations for the computation of a 1-D complex FFT that is proportional to $5N \log_2 N$. A more optimized variant has been published by [John 07]. Here, the number of required floating-point operations is only

$$N_{FFT} = \frac{34}{9} N \log_2 N - \frac{124}{27} N - 2 \log_2 N - \frac{2}{9}(-1)^{\log_2 N} \log_2 N + \frac{16}{27}(-1)^{\log_2 N} + 8 \tag{2.20}$$

for a convolution length of $N_{conv} = N$. Due to zero-padding N_{conv} is usually chosen such that $N_{conv} = 2N_u$. The complex multiplication in the frequency domain requires only two additions and two multiplications for each computed complex frequency value since the used filter kernels have either only real values or imaginary values in the frequency domain. As already mentioned in Section 2.2.2.1 it is possible to compute the Fourier-based convolution for two (real-valued) input vectors simultaneously using complex FFTs. Therefore,

$$N_{frequency} = N_{FFT} + 4 N_{conv} \tag{2.21}$$

floating-point operations are required for a single input vector resulting in a time complexity of $\mathcal{O}(N^3 \log_2 N)$ when $N = N_{conv} = N_u = N_v = N_p$.

Figure 2.3 shows the break-even points for various convolution length according to our analysis. Therefore, it is more efficient to implement a 1-D convolution in the frequency domain if filter mask sizes are larger than 19 pixels when $N_{conv} = 2048$ or 21 pixels when $N_{conv} = 4096$.

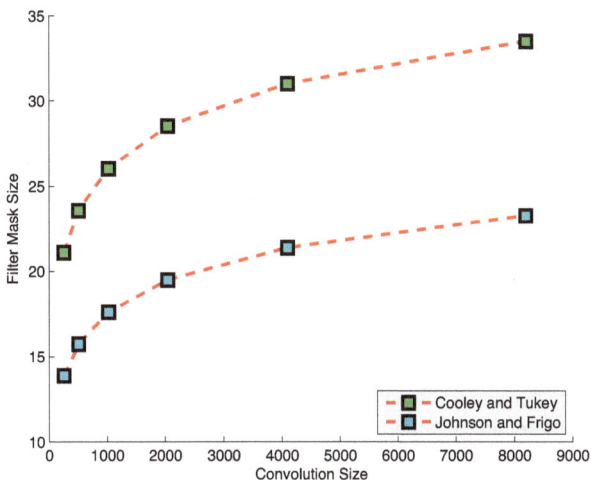

Figure 2.3: Comparison of computational efficiency for spatial- and frequency-based convolution filtering. The break-even point is given as the largest filter mask size where convolution filtering in the spatial domain is still superior than frequency-based convolution. When using larger filter mask sizes frequency-based convolution is more efficient. The break-even points are given for two well-known FFT implementations.

2.2.3.2 Back-Projection

The time complexity of back-projection is significantly higher. In our voxel-based approach it is necessary to compute the back-projection for each voxel of the volume ($N_{voxels} = N_x N_y N_z$) and each projection image N_p. The number of voxels in each direction usually equals the number of projection images ($N_x = N_y = N_z = N_p$). Therefore, the time complexity of back-projection is $\mathcal{O}(N^4)$.

The voxel-based back-projection according to Algorithm 1 requires for each voxel nine multiplications and nine additions to compute the matrix vector product, two multiplications and two divisions for the computation of the pixel coordinates (dehomogenize), two multiplications to apply the voxel-dependent distance weight, and one addition to add the computed voxel increment to the previous voxel value. Therefore, the back-projection of a single projection image requires

$$N_{Bp} = (24 + N_i)N_{voxels} \qquad (2.22)$$

floating-point operations. Here, N_i is the number of floating-point operations that are required for the interpolation when accessing the projection image (function fetch in Algorithm 1).

Nearest neighbor interpolation can be implemented by incrementing the computed coordinates $\breve{u}$ and $\breve{v}$ by 0.5 before they are truncated to integer numbers. This increment can be integrated into the projection matrix as a translation of the PCS, and

Algorithmic Step	Fraction of Computational Time
Pre-processing (without filtering)	5 %
Filtering	19 %
Back-projection	71 %
Post-processing	5 %

Table 2.1: Fractions of computational time in a practical cone-beam CT system for different processing steps. Table taken from [Heig 07].

thus $N_i = 0$ for nearest neighbor interpolation. However, for bilinear interpolation $N_i = 10$ (six additions and four multiplications). Note that some hardware architectures, e.g. graphics accelerators, implement this operation in hardware resulting in $N_i = 1$ or even $N_i = 0$.

The number of required floating-point operations can be significantly reduced when using the incremental version of Algorithm 2. By the incremental computation of the matrix vector product six multiplications and six additions are moved out of the innermost loop. Therefore, the back-projection of a single projection image now requires only

$$N_{BpIncr} = (12 + N_i)N_{voxels} + 6N_y N_z + 6N_z \qquad (2.23)$$

floating-point operations. Compared to Algorithm 1 this reduces the number of required floating-point operations by over 35% when $N_i = 10$ or by nearly 50% when $N_i = 0$.

2.2.3.3   Comparison of Computation Times

Heigl and Kowarschik presented a performance analysis considering all processing steps in a practical C-arm CT system [Heig 07]. They measured relative timings of each processing task on a single-core CPU for 543 projection images with 1240×960 pixels each and a volume consisting of $512 \times 512 \times 440$ voxels.

Table 2.1 shows the time fractions of the particular algorithmic steps. The pre-processing tasks include intensity and beam hardening correction, scatter estimation and correction, and truncation correction, while post-processing includes the suppression of ring artifacts, which are caused by detector gain inhomogeneities. The pre-processing and post-processing steps, which are not considered in this thesis, take only 10% of the overall processing time. Therefore, our evaluation of filtering and back-projection on different hardware acceleration platforms addresses over 90% of the computational burden in a typical cone-beam CT system.

2.3   Selected Alternatives to the Feldkamp Algorithm

2.3.1   The M-Line Method

In medical imaging a high image quality is required. In the state-of-the-art FDK method [Feld 84], however, the occurring cone artifacts may cover small object details complicating their distinction.

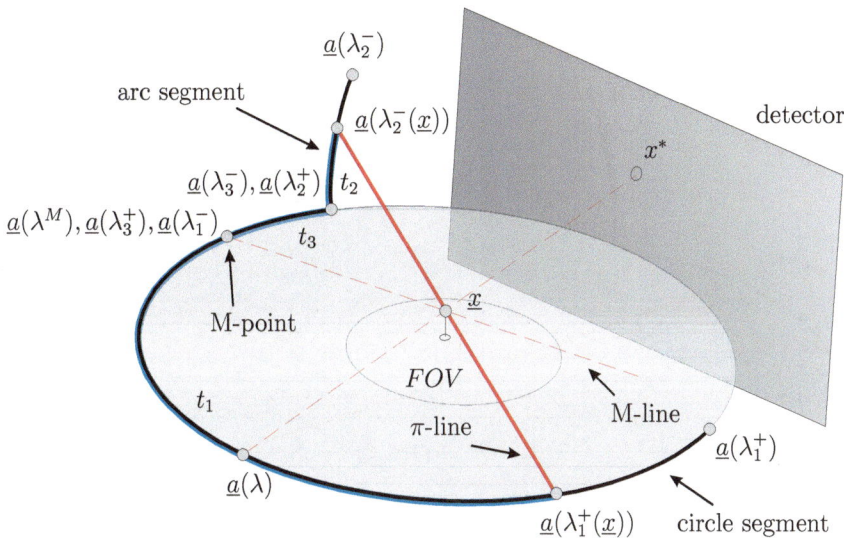

Figure 2.4: Geometry setup of the M-line reconstruction for the circle-plus-arc trajectory. For each point $\underline{x}$ to be reconstructed there exists exactly one M-line and one π-line. While the M-line defines the filtering lines (see also Figure 2.5), the π-line determines the source positions on the trajectory, where the cone-beam projections are back-projected onto $\underline{x}$.

Theoretically exact and stable cone-beam reconstruction algorithms (e.g., the M-line method [Pack 05]) provide excellent image quality without any cone artifacts. Although the M-line approach is still of a filtered back-projection style, it has an increased computational complexity as it requires additional computations for the filtering of the projection images; e.g., derivative computation and filtering along oblique lines in the projection. Thus, especially the filtering of projections incurs much more computations to be performed by the image reconstruction hardware.

The M-line approach can be applied for C-arm CT [Hopp 06]. It is, however, required that Tuy's data completeness condition for image reconstruction is fulfilled [Tuy 83]. According to Tuy it is possible to reconstruct the point $\underline{x}$ in a theoretically exact manner if and only if every plane through $\underline{x}$ intersects the source trajectory at least once. This intersection should not happen tangentially to the trajectory and not at an endpoint of the trajectory.

Due to the requirement of a complete cone-beam data acquisition, the source trajectory has to be extended. In our case we have chosen a short-scan circle-plus-arc acquisition where the source trajectory has been extended by an arc segment as shown in Figure 2.4. This extension is a practical choice for nearly all existent C-arm devices. Other trajectory extensions are also possible; e.g., the extension by a line segment.

The M-line method introduces a specific point on the source trajectory, called the M-point. In fact a different M-point could be selected for each point $\underline{x}$ within the

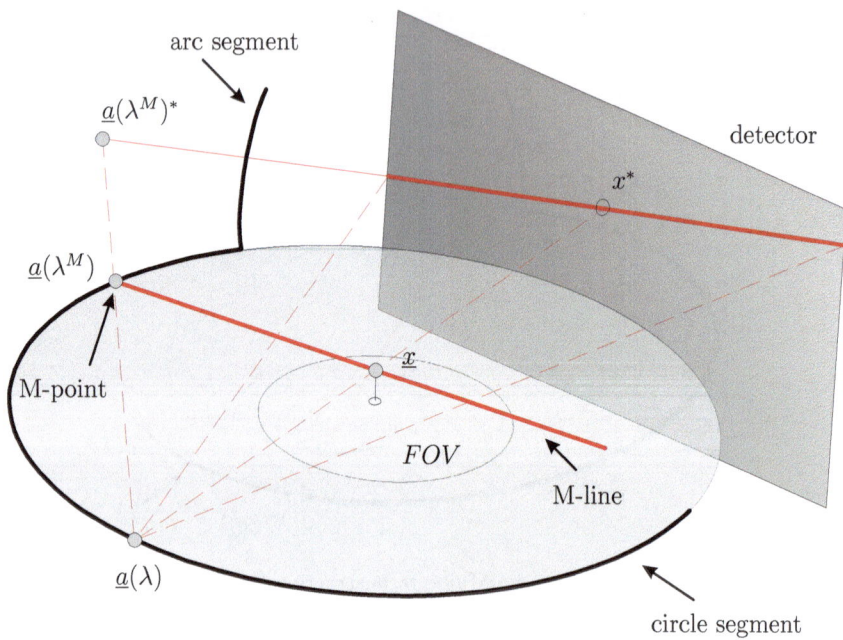

Figure 2.5: Derivation of the filtering line on the detector plane for point $\underline{x}$ during processing of the cone-beam projection corresponding to the source position at $\underline{a}(\lambda)$. The filtering line for $\underline{x}$ is given by the projection of its M-line onto the detector plane.

support of the object density function f. However, in order to achieve an efficient FBP formulation of the M-line approach, the M-point must be chosen fixed for each point $\underline{x}$ to be reconstructed. The M-point should further be selected such that it is (approximately) located in the middle of the circle segment [Hopp 06, Pack 05]. This choice reduces artifacts resulting from axial data truncation in case of long objects.

For each projection the M-line associated with the point $\underline{x}$ is defined as the line connecting the M-point with this point. As can be seen in Figure 2.5 the filtering line for $\underline{x}$ is then given by the projection of its M-line onto the detector plane. All points which are located in the plane defined by $\underline{a}(\lambda)$, $\underline{a}(\lambda^M)$, and $\underline{x}$ share the same filtering line. Thus, filtering can be done independently of $\underline{x}$ on a one-dimensional family of lines, prior to back-projection. This is a major advantage of the M-line method. It allows the reconstruction to be done in a computationally efficient FBP form.

Reconstruction using the M-line approach can only be achieved for points that are located on so called π-lines. A π-line is defined as a line connecting two different points on the source trajectory. For example, in Figure 2.4 the red line is the corresponding π-line of $\underline{x}$ connecting the point $\underline{a}(\lambda_1^+(\underline{x}))$ on the circle segment with the point $\underline{a}(\lambda_2^-(\underline{x}))$ on the arc segment. For the circle-plus-arc trajectory it is shown in [Kats 05] that each π-line is unique and that a large continuous volume is covered by π-lines. Similar results can be obtained for the circle-plus-line trajectory [Kats 04].

For each point $\underline{x}$ back-projection is carried out over three curve segments of the circle-plus-arc trajectory (see Figure 2.4). The first curve segment is located on the circle segment and goes from the selected M-point $\underline{a}(\lambda^M) = \underline{a}(\lambda_1^-)$ to the point $\underline{a}(\lambda_1^+(\underline{x}))$, which is the intersection point of the π-line containing $\underline{x}$ with the circle segment. The second curve segment reaches from the intersection point of the π-line with the arc segment $\underline{a}(\lambda_2^-(\underline{x}))$ to the foot point of the arc segment $\underline{a}(\lambda_2^+)$. Finally, the third curve segment is defined by the portion of the circle segment delimited by the foot point of the arc segment $\underline{a}(\lambda_3^-)$ and the selected M-point $\underline{a}(\lambda^M) = \underline{a}(\lambda_3^+)$.

In order to account for redundantly measured data, each of these segments is given a different weighting factor. While the first segment has weight 1, the other two segments are given a weighting factor of -1. This ensures a correct weighting of redundantly measured cone-beam data. Thus, the final reconstruction result is computed by subtracting the back-projection results of the last two segments from the back-projection result of the first segment. For a detailed derivation of the algorithm, we refer to [Pack 05].

2.3.1.1 Algorithmic Steps

To reconstruct a point $\underline{x}$ inside the support of the object with the M-line approach, the following steps are applied successively.

Step 1 – Filtering. Each projection $g(\lambda, \underline{\theta}(u, v))$ is turned into a filtered projection $g^F(\lambda, u, v)$ according to the following steps F1 to F6:

F1 – Derivative. Compute the derivative of $g(\lambda, \underline{\theta}(u, v))$ with respect to λ along a constant viewing direction $\underline{\theta}(u, v)$

$$g_1(\lambda, u, v) = \frac{\partial}{\partial \lambda} g(\lambda, \underline{\theta}(u, v)) \Big|_{\underline{\theta}(u,v)=\text{fixed}}, \tag{2.24}$$

with $\underline{\theta}(u, v)$ defined in Equation (2.2).

F2 – Cosine Weighting. Weight the data according to

$$g_2(\lambda, u, v) = \frac{D}{\sqrt{u^2 + v^2 + D^2}} g_1(\lambda, u, v). \tag{2.25}$$

F3 – Forward Rebinning (M-line specific). Perform a forward rebinning from detector coordinates $(u, v)^T$ to filtering line coordinates $(u, s)^T$, where s identifies the slope of the filtering line, according to

$$g_3(\lambda, u, s) = g_2(\lambda, u, v(u, s)), \tag{2.26}$$

where

$$v(u, s) = s(u - u_M) + v_M. \tag{2.27}$$

Here, all filtering lines converge to the projection of the common M-point $\underline{a}(\lambda^M)$ onto the detector. The projection $\underline{a}(\lambda^M)^*$ of the M-point is given by

$$\underline{a}(\lambda^M)^* = (u_M, v_M)^T. \tag{2.28}$$

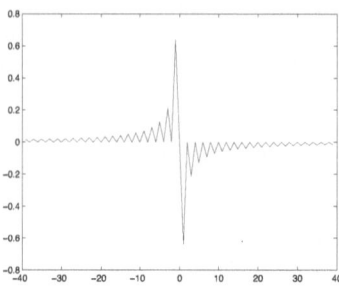 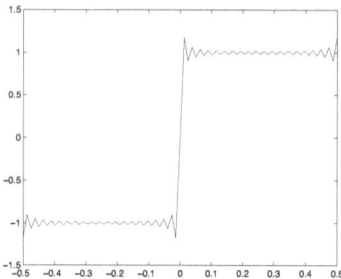

Figure 2.6:   Illustration of the Hilbert filter kernel. On the left side the impulse response of the Hilbert filter is shown. On the right side the ideal filter response is shown in the frequency domain. It has been band-limited to $1/(2\,du)$. Here, du denotes the width of a pixel in direction $\underline{e}_u$.

Consequently, each filtering line is uniquely identified by its slope and the mapping is invertible. After forward rebinning each row of the rebinned detector holds the values for exactly one filtering line.

F4 – Hilbert Filtering.   Perform a one-dimensional Hilbert transform (see Figure 2.6) with respect to u by computing

$$g_4(\lambda, u, s) = \int_{-\infty}^{+\infty} \frac{1}{\pi(u - u')} g_3(\lambda, u', s) du' . \tag{2.29}$$

F5 – Backward Rebinning (M-line specific).   In order to achieve a computationally more efficient back-projection, we avoid the direct back-projection from the rebinned grid. Instead we perform a backward rebinning from filtering line coordinates $(u, s)^T$ to detector coordinates $(u, v)^T$ according to

$$g_5(\lambda, u, v) = g_4(\lambda, u, s(u, v)) , \tag{2.30}$$

where

$$s(u, v) = \frac{v - v_M}{u - u_M} . \tag{2.31}$$

F6 – π-line Weighting.   Perform π-line weighting according to

$$g^F(\lambda, u, v) = m(\lambda, u, v) g_5(\lambda, u, v) . \tag{2.32}$$

The function $m(\lambda, u, v)$ takes only values of zero or one and should be understood as a 2-D weighting mask that accounts for a correct handling of the back-projection segments for each point $\underline{x}$. It can be precomputed once after C-arm geometry calibration as shown in [Hopp 06] (Section VI).

The decision if the current source position is inside the back-projection interval for a point $\underline{x}$ can be made either by projecting the circle segment to the detector when the source is on the arc segment or by projecting the arc segment to the detector when the source is on the circle segment (see Figure 2.7). Assume the source position moves along the circle segment. Then the current source position is inside the back-projection interval corresponding to point $\underline{x}$ when $\underline{x}$ projects to the right-hand side of the projected arc segment. If $\underline{x}$ projects to the left-hand side of the arc segment the current source position is outside of the back-projection interval. This is true for every point on the line connecting the current source position and point $\underline{x}$. It follows that mask values depend only on the projection of $\underline{x}$ onto the detector. It is therefore justified to create a 2-D weighting mask $m(\lambda, u, v)$, which assigns each detector point $(u, v)^T$ on the right-hand side a value of one, and a value of zero otherwise. The same principle applies if the source moves along the arc segment. In this case the current source position is inside the back-projection interval corresponding to point $\underline{x}$ when $\underline{x}$ projects above the projected circle segment. Here, the weighting mask $m(\lambda, u, v)$ assigns each detector point $(u, v)^T$ on top of the projected circle segment a value of one, and a value of zero otherwise.

Step 2 – Back-Projection. Back-project the filtered projection $g^F(\lambda, u, v)$ into the image space to obtain f at each point $\underline{x} = (x, y, z)^T$ according to

$$f(\underline{x}) = -\frac{1}{2\pi^2} \sum_{q=1}^{3} t_q \int_{\lambda_q^-}^{\lambda_q^+} \frac{1}{|\langle(\underline{x} - \underline{a}(\lambda)), \underline{e}_w\rangle|} g^F(\lambda, u(\lambda, \underline{x}), v(\lambda, \underline{x})) d\lambda, \qquad (2.33)$$

where u and v are the detector coordinates corresponding to $\underline{x}$ and λ, given by

$$u(\lambda, \underline{x}) = -D\frac{\langle(\underline{x} - \underline{a}(\lambda)), \underline{e}_u\rangle}{\langle(\underline{x} - \underline{a}(\lambda)), \underline{e}_w\rangle}, \qquad (2.34)$$

$$v(\lambda, \underline{x}) = -D\frac{\langle(\underline{x} - \underline{a}(\lambda)), \underline{e}_v\rangle}{\langle(\underline{x} - \underline{a}(\lambda)), \underline{e}_w\rangle}, \qquad (2.35)$$

and $t_1 = 1$, $t_2 = -1$, $t_3 = -1$; cf. Figure 2.4. The back-projection segments for each point $\underline{x}$ are already handled by the multiplication with the π-line weighting mask $m(\lambda, u, v)$ in filtering step F6. Therefore, in Equation (2.33) we really used λ_1^+ and λ_2^- corresponding to the endpoints of the trajectory as the back-projection interval limits instead of $\lambda_1^+(\underline{x})$ and $\lambda_2^-(\underline{x})$ for the first two segments, respectively. This has the advantage that the different back-projection intervals do not depend on the point $\underline{x}$ to be reconstructed. Because other exact cone-beam reconstruction algorithms (e.g., [Kats 05]) can be implemented in a similar way, M-line specific steps have been marked as such. As can be seen only the rebinning steps have to be modified in order to account for other filtering directions.

2.3.1.2 Implementation Strategies

Derivative. The M-line method requires the computation of a view-dependent derivative of the following form

$$\frac{\partial}{\partial \lambda} g(\lambda, \underline{\theta})\bigg|_{\underline{\theta}=\text{fixed}} = \lim_{\epsilon \to 0} \frac{g(\lambda + \epsilon, \underline{\theta}) - g(\lambda - \epsilon, \underline{\theta})}{2\epsilon} \qquad (2.36)$$

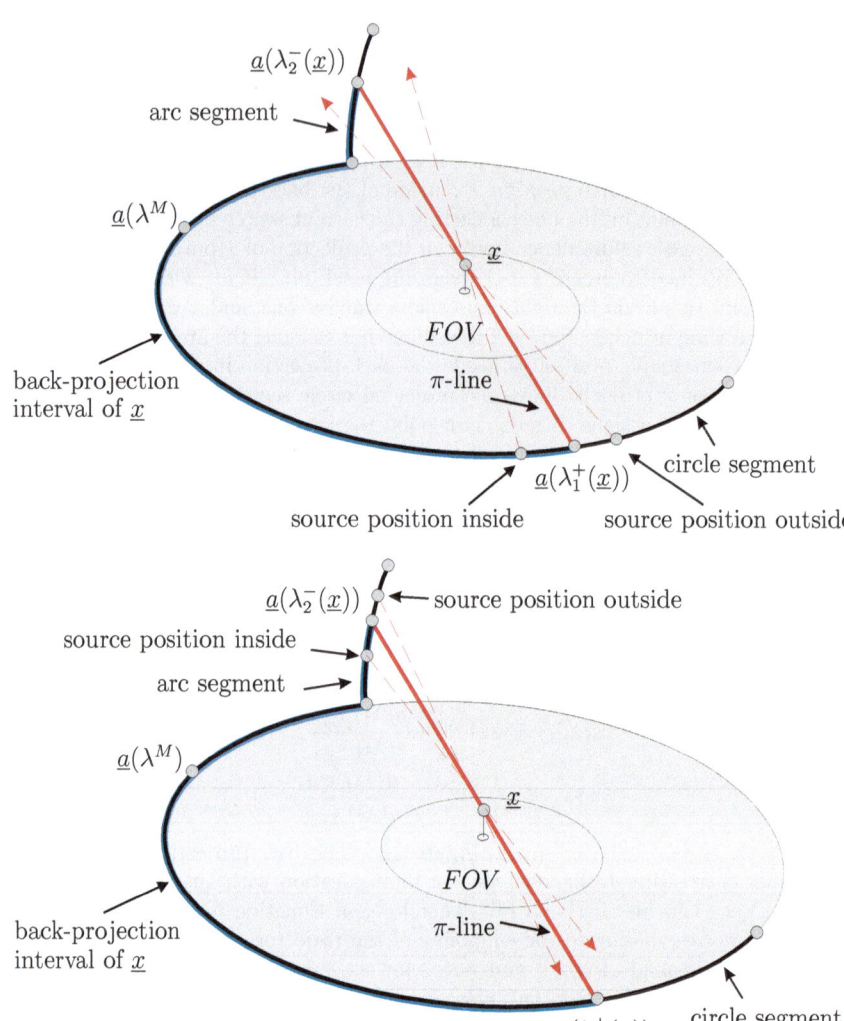

Figure 2.7:   Illustration of π-line weighting. When the source is on the circle segment (top) the source is within the back-projection interval (shown in bold blue) corresponding to the point $\underline{x}$ only if $\underline{x}$ projects to the right hand side of the projected arc segment. Otherwise $\underline{x}$ projects to the left hand side of the projected arc segment. When the source is on the arc segment (bottom) the source is within the back-projection interval corresponding to the point $\underline{x}$ only if $\underline{x}$ projects above the projected circle segment. Otherwise $\underline{x}$ projects below the projected circle segment.

as a first-processing step (see Equation (2.24)). Basically, $g(\lambda, \underline{\theta})$ has to be differentiated with respect to λ while keeping the ray direction $\underline{\theta} = \underline{\theta}(u, v)$ fixed. It is difficult to implement this formula accurately because the sampled values of $\underline{\theta}$ change with λ as they are specified by the detector sampling and the position of the source and detector relative to each other. Furthermore, the sampling in λ is often coarser than the sampling on the detector. The chain-rule can be applied to the view-dependent derivative as follows

$$\frac{\partial}{\partial\lambda}g(\lambda, \underline{\theta}(u,v))\Big|_{\underline{\theta}(u,v)=\text{fixed}} = \frac{\partial}{\partial\lambda}g(\lambda, \underline{\theta})\Big|_{\underline{\theta}=\text{fixed}} = \left(\frac{\partial g}{\partial\lambda} + \frac{\partial g}{\partial u}\frac{\partial u}{\partial\lambda} + \frac{\partial g}{\partial v}\frac{\partial v}{\partial\lambda}\right) \quad (2.37)$$

with u and v given by

$$u = -D\frac{\langle\underline{\theta}, \underline{e}_u(\lambda)\rangle}{\langle\underline{\theta}, \underline{e}_w\rangle}, \quad (2.38)$$

$$v = -D\frac{\langle\underline{\theta}, \underline{e}_v(\lambda)\rangle}{\langle\underline{\theta}, \underline{e}_w\rangle}. \quad (2.39)$$

It can be seen that only the first term in Equation (2.37) requires the differentiation with respect to λ. Compared to a straightforward implementation this approach often yields a much higher resolution [Noo 03].

Replacing u and v by the expressions in Equations (2.38) and (2.39), respectively, we further get

$$\frac{\partial u}{\partial\lambda}\Big|_{\underline{\theta}=\text{fixed}} = \frac{-D(\langle\underline{\theta}, \underline{e}'_u(\lambda)\rangle \cdot \langle\underline{\theta}, \underline{e}_w(\lambda)\rangle - \langle\underline{\theta}, \underline{e}_u(\lambda)\rangle \cdot \langle\underline{\theta}, \underline{e}'_w(\lambda)\rangle)}{\langle\underline{\theta}, \underline{e}_w(\lambda)\rangle^2}, \quad (2.40)$$

$$\frac{\partial v}{\partial\lambda}\Big|_{\underline{\theta}=\text{fixed}} = \frac{-D(\langle\underline{\theta}, \underline{e}'_v(\lambda)\rangle \cdot \langle\underline{\theta}, \underline{e}_w(\lambda)\rangle - \langle\underline{\theta}, \underline{e}_v(\lambda)\rangle \cdot \langle\underline{\theta}, \underline{e}'_w(\lambda)\rangle)}{\langle\underline{\theta}, \underline{e}_w(\lambda)\rangle^2}. \quad (2.41)$$

Here, we assumed in favor of a computationally more efficient implementation that D does not depend on λ, which may not be guaranteed in a non-ideal acquisition but practically introduces only a marginal error in the final result.

Using Equation (2.37) the computation of the view-dependent derivative of a projection image can thus be discretized and implemented according to Algorithm 3. In this algorithm we used the following equality

$$\frac{\|\underline{\theta}\|_2}{\langle\underline{\theta}, \underline{e}_w(\lambda)\rangle^2} = \frac{u^2 + v^2 + D^2}{D}, \quad (2.42)$$

and the source-detector distance D, the unit vectors $\underline{e}_u(\lambda)$, $\underline{e}_v(\lambda)$, and $\underline{e}_w(\lambda)$ are extracted from the corresponding projection matrix $\mathbf{P}(\lambda)$ using the function "extractGeometry".[5] All derivatives are discretized using central differences, i.e. the derivative $h'(x)$ of a function $h(x)$ is numerically computed according to

$$h'(x) \simeq \frac{h(x+\epsilon) - h(x-\epsilon)}{2\epsilon} \quad (2.43)$$

with ϵ chosen according to the sampling interval of that function. Algorithm 3 can be used to compute the derivative adequately in practical acquisitions that deviate slightly from an ideal scan geometry.

---

[5] See Appendix A how the function "extractGeometry" can be implemented to extract the geometrical parameters from a projection matrix.

Algorithm 3: Computation of the view-dependent derivative of a projection image.

Input: Three successive projection images $\mathbf{I}_i$, $0 \leq i < 3$, having $N_u \times N_v$ pixels each

Input: Corresponding projection matrices $\mathbf{P}_i$, $0 \leq i < 3$

Input: Pixel size du and dv

Input: Average distance $d\lambda$ between two source positions on the trajectory

Result: View-dependent derivative $\mathbf{I}'$ of projection image $\mathbf{I}_1$

```
// Extract geometrical parameters
```

1　$\left[\ \underline{e}_{u0}\ \ \underline{e}_{v0}\ \ \underline{e}_{w0}\ \ u_{00}\ \ v_{00}\ \ D_0\ \right] = \text{extractGeometry}(\mathbf{P}_0, du, dv)$;

2　$\left[\ \underline{e}_{u1}\ \ \underline{e}_{v1}\ \ \underline{e}_{w1}\ \ u_{01}\ \ v_{01}\ \ D_1\ \right] = \text{extractGeometry}(\mathbf{P}_1, du, dv)$;

3　$\left[\ \underline{e}_{u2}\ \ \underline{e}_{v2}\ \ \underline{e}_{w2}\ \ u_{02}\ \ v_{02}\ \ D_2\ \right] = \text{extractGeometry}(\mathbf{P}_2, du, dv)$;

4　**for** $(\check{v} = 0; \check{v} < N_v; \check{v} = \check{v} + 1)$ **do**

5　　**for** $(\check{u} = 0; \check{u} < N_u; \check{u} = \check{u} + 1)$ **do**

```
      // Compute detector coordinates
```

6　　　$u = (\check{u} - u_{01})du$;

7　　　$v = (\check{v} - v_{01})dv$;

```
      // Compute normalized direction vector
```

8　　　$f = u^2 + v^2 + D_1^2$;

9　　　$\theta = (u\underline{e}_{u1} - D_1\underline{e}_{w1} + v\underline{e}_{v1})/sqrt(f)$;

```
      // Compute derivatives
```

10　　　$\frac{\partial g}{\partial \lambda} = (\mathbf{I}_2[\check{u}, \check{v}] - \mathbf{I}_0[\check{u}, \check{v}])/(2\,d\lambda)$;

11　　　$\underline{e}'_u = (\underline{e}_{u2} - \underline{e}_{u0})/(2d\lambda)$;

12　　　$\underline{e}'_v = (\underline{e}_{v2} - \underline{e}_{v0})/(2d\lambda)$;

13　　　$\underline{e}'_w = (\underline{e}_{w2} - \underline{e}_{w0})/(2d\lambda)$;

14　　　$\frac{\partial u}{\partial \lambda} = -f(\langle \underline{\theta}, \underline{e}'_u \rangle \cdot \langle \underline{\theta}, \underline{e}_{w1} \rangle - \langle \underline{\theta}, \underline{e}_{u1} \rangle \cdot \langle \underline{\theta}, \underline{e}'_w \rangle)/D_1$;

15　　　$\frac{\partial v}{\partial \lambda} = -f(\langle \underline{\theta}, \underline{e}'_v \rangle \cdot \langle \underline{\theta}, \underline{e}_{w1} \rangle - \langle \underline{\theta}, \underline{e}_{v1} \rangle \cdot \langle \underline{\theta}, \underline{e}'_w \rangle)/D_1$;

16　　　$\frac{\partial g}{\partial u} = (\mathbf{I}_1[\check{u} + 1, \check{v}] - \mathbf{I}_1[\check{u} - 1, \check{v}])/(2D_1)$;

17　　　$\frac{\partial g}{\partial v} = (\mathbf{I}_1[\check{u}, \check{v} + 1] - \mathbf{I}_1[\check{u}, \check{v} - 1])/(2D_1)$;

18　　　$\mathbf{I}'[\check{u}, \check{v}] = \frac{\partial g}{\partial \lambda} + \frac{\partial g}{\partial u}\frac{\partial u}{\partial \lambda} + \frac{\partial g}{\partial v}\frac{\partial v}{\partial \lambda}$;

19　　**end**

20　**end**

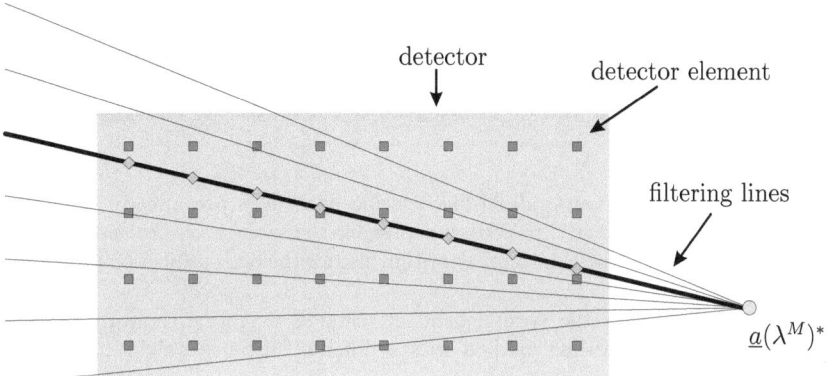

Figure 2.8: Forward rebinning: the values of the filtering line coordinates (diamonds) are computed by linear interpolation from the values of the original detector grid (squares). Because the sampling in horizontal direction coincides between the filtering lines and the detector grid, interpolation is only necessary in vertical direction.

Rebinning. The values of the filtering line coordinates according to the forward rebinning step (F3) are computed such that interpolation needs to be done only in v-direction. Therefore we choose the sampling points of the filtering line coordinates to coincide with the original detector coordinates in u-direction (see Figure 2.8).

The projection of the M-point $\underline{a}(\lambda^M)^*$ onto the detector is computed using the corresponding projection matrix $\mathbf{P}(\lambda)$. The homogeneous representation of the projection of the M-point is thus given by the matrix vector product of the projection matrix and the M-point. This approach easily incorporates any necessary modifications of the rebinning formula in a non-ideal acquisition.

The backward rebinning operations according to filtering step (F5) are computed using the implementation strategy that is used during forward rebinning in reversed order.

π-Line Weighting. In order to compute the π-line weighting mask $m(\lambda, u, v)$ we project the source positions of the respective source trajectory, where projection images are acquired, onto the detector plane. Each source position along the arc segment is projected when the current source position is on the circle segment, otherwise each source position along the circle segment is projected. Then, we remove all projected points that are not within the defined detector boundaries and extrapolate the resulting polygonal curve to the detector boundaries. The mask values (zero or one) are computed according to the polygonal curve representation of the projected trajectory segment as already outlined in Section 2.3.1.1 (Filtering Step F6). If less than two points project within the detector boundaries a value of one is assigned to each pixel of the weighting mask.

Finally, we generate a smooth transition zone within a small neighborhood of the polygonal curve in order to avoid artifacts along the π-lines in the final reconstruction.

This is done by applying a one-dimensional convolution of the weighting mask with a simple averaging filter in row direction when the source is on the circle segment and in column direction when the source is on the line segment. We selected a filter mask size of three pixels, which provided good results at least for our specific C-arm geometry.

Back-Projection. Because all M-line specific operations are already computed during the filtering steps (F1) to (F6), it is possible to use the back-projection implementation approach of the Feldkamp algorithm also for the back-projection processing in the M-line method.

The computation of the voxel-dependent distance weighting, however, had to be changed since the M-line method uses a different distance weight (cf. Equation (2.33)):

$$\mu_{Mline}(\lambda, \underline{x}) = \frac{1}{|\langle(\underline{x} - \underline{a}(\lambda)), \underline{e}_w\rangle|}. \tag{2.44}$$

From Equation (2.17) follows that the distance weight of the M-line method can be computed by $-s/t$ rather than by $1/t^2$:

$$\mu_{Mline}(\lambda, \underline{x}) = -s\frac{\sqrt{R^2}}{\sqrt{\langle(\underline{x} - \underline{a}(\lambda)), \underline{e}_w\rangle^2}} = -s\sqrt{\mu_{FDK}(\lambda, \underline{x})} = -s\frac{1}{t} \tag{2.45}$$

with $s = -\frac{1}{R}$, where R is the distance between the source and the rotation axis. The minus sign results from the direction of $\underline{e}_w$, which points from the origin of the DCS towards the source position.

In non-ideal acquisitions R depends on λ and thus the factor $s = s(\lambda)$ must be calculated from

$$s(\lambda) = \frac{1}{\|\underline{a}(\lambda)\|_2} \tag{2.46}$$

for each source position. The vector $\underline{a}(\lambda)$ can be extracted from the projection matrix (see Appendix A). The scaling by the factor s can be efficiently computed during filtering step (F4) by scaling the values of the filter kernel accordingly.

2.3.2   Iterative Reconstruction

The 3-D image reconstruction task can also be solved using an entirely different approach. The problem can be formulated as a large-scale system of linear equations where the linear attenuation coefficients are the unknowns and each measured line integral adds an additional equation to the system. Due to the large size of the considered linear systems iterative methods such as the algebraic reconstruction technique (ART) are usually applied in order to solve the reconstruction problem.

While this approach is conceptually simpler than analytical approaches it has a higher computational complexity. However, iterative methods show improved image quality when it is not feasible or simply not desired to measure a sufficiently large number of projections. Iterative approaches further achieve better image quality when the projections are not uniformly distributed over the scan trajectory [Kak 01, Muel 98].

In the following we provide the theoretical foundations of the simultaneous algebraic reconstruction technique (SART) and focus on implementation choices of the most time-consuming parts of the algorithm. For a detailed overview of algebraic reconstruction techniques we refer to [Kak 01]. A detailed comparison of iterative reconstruction algorithms can be found in [Zhan 06]. In the following we adopt their notation.

2.3.2.1 Simultaneous Algebraic Reconstruction Technique

The ART method was proposed in [Gord 70] for the reconstruction of three-dimensional objects from electron-microscopic scans and X-ray photography. The reconstruction volume is subdivided into J voxels where the jth voxel is denoted by x_j, $0 \leq j < J$. We assume that in each voxel x_j the function of the linear attenuation coefficient is constant. Each projection image contains I elements. The ith ray, $0 \leq i < I$, is defined as the line segment starting from the x-ray source position to the center of the ith detector element of that projection. Consider the nth projection from the total number N of measured projections, $0 \leq n < N$. Let the path length of the ith ray of the nth projection going through the jth voxel be denoted by $a_{ij,n}$. Then, we can formulate for each projection view n a system of linear equations in terms of the measured projection data $y_{i,n}$:

$$\sum_{j=0}^{J-1} a_{ij,n} x_j = y_{i,n} \quad , \quad 0 \leq i < I . \tag{2.47}$$

Here, each $y_{i,n}$ corresponds to a measured line integral $g(\lambda, \underline{\theta}(u, v))$. We can rewrite Equation (2.47) in matrix vector form as

$$\mathbf{A}_n \underline{x} = \underline{y}_n , \tag{2.48}$$

where $\mathbf{A}_n = (a_{ij,n})_{0 \leq i < I, 0 \leq j < J}$ is the system matrix for the nth projection, $\underline{x}$ is the vector of unknown attenuation coefficients, and $\underline{y}_n$ is the vector of measured line integrals for the nth projection. The final linear system is obtained when the individual systems of linear equations for each projection view are stacked together:

$$\begin{bmatrix} \mathbf{A}_0 \\ \vdots \\ \mathbf{A}_{N-1} \end{bmatrix} \underline{x} = \begin{bmatrix} \underline{y}_0 \\ \vdots \\ \underline{y}_{N-1} \end{bmatrix} \rightarrow \mathbf{A} \underline{x} = \underline{y} . \tag{2.49}$$

Since the size of matrix $\mathbf{A}$ is very large for practical reconstruction problems iterative methods are applied in order to solve the system of linear equations. Using the Kaczmarz method [Kacz 37] the reconstruction is accomplished by iteratively updating the unknown linear attenuation coefficients $\underline{x}$ in a "ray-by-ray" manner. In each update step a forward-projection through the current voxel volume along the ray under consideration is computed, and in the following back-projection step the voxels, which are affected by the ray, are updated by the difference between the computed line integral and the measured line integral. This difference contributes to each voxel according to the proportion of the path length of the ray inside the voxel and the complete path length of the ray through the volume.

Using highly parallel computing hardware it is nearly impossible to efficiently implement iterative reconstruction algorithms, which require voxel updates in a "ray-by-ray" manner. Fortunately there are other formulations of ART, which are better suited for an efficient parallel implementation and at the same time have even better noise properties [Muel 98].

The simultaneous algebraic reconstruction technique (SART) updates the voxel volume simultaneously after all rays of a projection image have been processed. This allows to efficiently compute the forward-projection and the back-projection along the rays of each projection in parallel.

In the following we describe the update formula for the SART method. In each iteration of the SART method all projections N are processed. The processing order of the projections strongly influences the practical performance of the method. It has been suggested that the information of two successively processed projections should be correlated as less as possible [Guan 94]. During processing we define the approximation of the linear attenuation coefficient for the jth voxel as $\hat{x}_j^{k,n}$. The index k denotes how many iterations have been completed so far. The index n denotes how many projections have previously been processed in iteration k and thus how many simultaneous voxel update steps have been done during that iteration step. The starting value of the jth voxel in iteration $k + 1$ is defined as $\hat{x}_j^{k+1,0} = \hat{x}_j^{k,N}$.

If we denote by $M_{j,n}$ the total number of rays in the nth projection going through the jth voxel, the update formula of SART for the jth voxel can be written as [Zhan 06]:

$$
\hat{x}_j^{k+1,n} = \hat{x}_j^{k+1,n-1} + \tau \frac{\displaystyle\sum_{m=0}^{M_{j,n}-1} a_{mj,n} \left(\frac{y_{m,n} - \displaystyle\sum_{j=0}^{J-1} a_{mj,n}\hat{x}_j^{k+1,n-1}}{\displaystyle\sum_{j=0}^{J-1} a_{mj,n}} \right)}{\displaystyle\sum_{m=0}^{M_{j,n}-1} a_{mj,n}} . \tag{2.50}
$$

Here m denotes the index of the subset $M_{j,n}$ of the I rays in the nth projection view. τ is a relaxation parameter, which is a small positive number (less than 1). It is used to reduce noise effects introduced by the update process.

There are several possibilities to choose the initial voxel values $\hat{x}_j^{0,0}$. They are often initialized to zero or very small positive values. Another option would be to initialize them to the result of other reconstruction approaches; e.g., the FDK method or simply the result of an unfiltered back-projection step. Streak artifacts appearing around high-contrast structures disappear very slowly with the iterations when the initial voxel volume is uniformly initialized. These artifacts are rapidly suppressed when an initial FDK reconstruction is used as a starting point at the expense of the injection of additional noise. This noise is, however, effectively removed after five to ten iterations [Zbij 03].

2.3.2.2   Implementation Strategies

The SART update formula (Equation (2.50)) consists mainly of two computationally expensive steps: forward-projection and back-projection. Both of them exhibit a sufficient large amount of operations, which can be computed highly efficiently on special hardware architectures.

In order to make use of the parallelism offered by these architectures the forward-projection step can be easily implemented in a ray-driven manner. Each sampled ray sum $0 \leq i < I$ can be computed in parallel.

Usually, the forward-projection is defined as the transposed operator of the back-projection. This leads to a ray-driven back-projection. However, we suggest to implement the back-projection step in a voxel-driven manner. Compared to a ray-driven back-projection implementation this approach is free of race conditions during the voxel updates. Furthermore, this implementation approach has another significant advantage because it avoids any computational operations, which are necessary to calculate the weighting coefficients of matrix $\mathbf{A}$ during back-projection. This is true because the size of the subset $M_{j,n}$ for each voxel j is exactly one in a voxel-driven back-projection implementation. It can be seen from Equation (2.50) that the sums over m are removed and the remaining weighting factors $a_{mj,n}$ in the numerator and the denominator are canceled out.

This results in the following simplified update formula for a voxel-driven back-projection implementation:

$$\hat{x}_j^{k+1,n} = \hat{x}_j^{k+1,n-1} + \tau \frac{y_{m,n} - \sum_{j=0}^{J-1} a_{mj,n} \hat{x}_j^{k+1,n-1}}{l_m} . \tag{2.51}$$

Here, m refers to the ray in projection n going through the center of voxel j and

$$l_m = \sum_{j=0}^{J-1} a_{mj,n} \tag{2.52}$$

is the path length of this ray through the complete volume. It must be stated that the ray m does not necessarily need to be included in the digitally sampled rays I of the considered projection n. This results from the implementation choice of a non-matching[6] forward-projection and back-projection pair. Forward-projection is computed ray-driven, back-projection voxel-driven. During back-projection all accesses to the differences of the projection values and the computed ray sums, which have not been computed during forward-projection are interpolated using the computed neighboring differences of the projection value and the computed ray sums of that projection. For example bilinear interpolation can be used for that.

The influence of a non-matching forward-projection and back-projection pair in the implementation of iterative reconstruction is investigated in [Zeng 00]. The authors conclude that using a matched or unmatched forward- and back-projection pair is not a very critical factor in a practical image reconstruction problem. An unmatched pair can even remove ring artifacts, which are otherwise introduced in reconstructions using a matched pair.

---

[6] Generally the term non-matching refers to the property that the forward-projection operator and the back-projection operator are not transposed of each other.

2.3.2.3 Other Iterative Algorithms

There are other variants of iterative reconstruction algorithms. The simultaneous iterative reconstruction technique (SIRT) is a variation of SART. It distinguishes from SART mainly because the voxels of the volume are only updated after all projections have been processed. Iterative FBP approaches are similar to SART or SIRT. In each update step, however, a ramp filter is applied to the difference images, which speeds up the convergence.

Using statistical iterative reconstruction algorithms (e.g., MLEM [Shep 82] or OSEM [Huds 94]) physical effects can be incorporated in order to achieve better image quality for noisy data. They have been successfully applied in molecular imaging scanners for a few years, for example.

While the theoretical formulations of iterative reconstruction algorithms may vary significantly, the most time-consuming parts remain to be the forward-projection through the voxel-volume and the back-projection of the difference images. For some algorithm variants (e.g., in statistical iterative approaches) these steps have to be applied even several times per update step.

We do not implement a complete iterative method in this thesis. Rather than that we focus on an efficient hardware implementation of the forward- and back-projection step. Doing it this way an estimate of the overall reconstruction time of a specific iterative reconstruction algorithm is easily possible.

2.4 Summary

We have presented three different approaches to solve the 3-D reconstruction task in medical imaging. The most common used reconstruction algorithm in practical cone-beam CT scanners is the FDK method. We have outlined the challenges to implement this algorithm for real CT systems that usually deviate slightly from the ideal Feldkamp geometry. Commonly a calibration step is performed in order to deal with such non-ideal acquisitions. We have derived an implementation approach that takes these deviations into account and is still amenable to a parallel implementation on high performance architectures. Finally, we have performed an analysis of the time complexity of the two most computationally expensive processing steps; the filtering of the image rows with time complexity $\mathcal{O}(N^3 \log_2 N)$, which constitutes roughly 20% of the overall computation time, and the back-projection step with time complexity $\mathcal{O}(N^4)$, which takes over 70% of the overall processing time in practical cone-beam CT systems.

Since the FDK method is of an approximative nature, its reconstruction results suffer from severe artifacts in certain situations. We have selected two alternative approaches to cone-beam reconstruction, which are able to deliver significantly improved image quality when compared to the results of the FDK method.

In this regard we have discussed the M-line method, which is a theoretically exact and stable reconstruction algorithm. The M-line method takes advantage from an extension of the source trajectory that guarantees a complete cone-beam data acquisition. Using this approach the problem of cone artifacts of FDK reconstructions is totally resolved. Additionally, we have presented an iterative reconstruction approach with a strong focus on its most time-consuming processing steps; the forward-projection and the back-projection.

Finally, we have derived appropriate implementation approaches, that are able to handle the non-ideal acquisitions in practical cone-beam CT systems, both for the M-line method and for iterative reconstruction methods.

Chapter 3

Design and Implementation of a General Reconstruction Framework

The design and implementation of the reconstruction system in medical X-ray imaging is a challenging issue due to its immense computational demands. In order to ensure an efficient clinical workflow it is inevitable to meet high performance requirements. Hence, the usage of hardware acceleration is mandatory. The software architecture of the reconstruction system is required to be modular in a sense that different accelerator hardware platforms are supported. It must be possible to implement different parts of the algorithm using different acceleration architectures and techniques.

This chapter introduces and discusses the design of a software architecture for an image reconstruction system that meets the aforementioned requirements. We implemented a multi-threaded software framework that combines three software design patterns: the pipeline, the master/worker [Matt 05], and the factory design pattern [Gamm 94]. This enables us to take advantage of the parallelism in off-the-shelf accelerator hardware such as multi-core systems, the Cell processor, and graphics accelerators in a very flexible and reusable way.

The main contributions of this chapter have been presented at the International Conference on Software Engineering 2008 [Sche 08].

3.1 Motivation

Scanning devices in medical imaging acquire a huge amount of data, e.g. X-ray projection images from different angles around the patient. Modern C-arm devices, for instance, generate more than 2 GigaByte (GB) of projection data for volume reconstruction. The basic computational structure of a reconstruction system consists of a series of processing tasks on these data, which finally results in the reconstructed volume, consisting of many transaxial slices through the patient.

The typical medical workflow – especially for interventional imaging using C-arm devices – requires high-speed reconstruction in order to avoid a delay of patient treatment during surgery, for example. Therefore, future practical reconstruction systems may present the reconstructed volume to the physician in real-time, immediately after the last projection image has been acquired by the scanning device. This requires to do all computations on-the-fly, which means that the reconstruction must be done in parallel to the data acquisition.

Our proposed software architecture is based upon a combination of parallel design patterns [Matt 05]. The main part of the reconstruction system follows the pipeline pattern [Posn 96, Verm 95] in order to organize the different processing tasks on the input data in concurrently executing stages. Achieving the objective to meet the immense computational demands on the reconstruction system, hardware acceleration of the respective processing tasks must be used in addition to the pipeline design. According to our experience parallel hardware architectures can be used most efficiently by following either the pipeline design pattern or the master/worker design pattern [Matt 05] in order to parallelize the computations of the respective pipeline stages.

Another advantage of our approach is its role as a hardware abstraction layer. The master/worker concept allows to abstract from the respective hardware accelerator used in a specific pipeline stage. In combination with the factory[1] design pattern [Alex 01, Gamm 94] most parts of the reconstruction algorithm can be expressed independently from the used acceleration hardware. The respective architecture execution configuration of the pipeline stages can even be changed dynamically at run-time.

We have done a thorough evaluation of the proposed design approach by implementing several reconstruction systems using the aforementioned hardware platforms (see Chapters 5 to 7). While the basic building parts as described by the combination of the pipeline and the master/worker design patterns remain the same for all reconstruction systems, we implemented this design paradigm using a multi-threaded approach in a software framework called *Reconstruction Toolkit* (RTK). The framework further addresses resource usage issues when allocating objects in the pipeline, e.g. the allocation and management of buffers for input data.

In the following section we briefly describe a state-of-the-art reconstruction system using an example of reconstruction in CT with C-arm devices. Then, we comment on the technical facts of the considered hardware architectures used to implement accelerated versions of such a system. In Section 3.2 we discuss in detail the design of a reconstruction system, which faces all important building blocks of its software architecture: the reconstruction pipeline (3.2.1), the parallelization strategy (3.2.2) and the resource management (3.2.3). The following section reflects the practical challenge in implementing the design in a software framework that is flexible, reusable, and easy to extend.

3.1.1   Cone-Beam CT Reconstruction

In this section we briefly recapitulate the computational steps involved in a state-of-the-art CT reconstruction system (e.g. a C-arm CT device) that is based upon the FDK reconstruction method [Feld 84].

---

[1] The factory design pattern provides an interface for creating families of related or dependent objects without specifying their concrete classes. This interface can then be implemented differently for a specific hardware configuration.

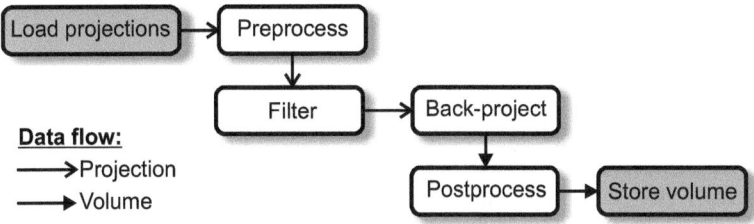

Figure 3.1: Processing steps of a state-of-the-art CT reconstruction system.

The reconstruction process can be subdivided into several parts [Heig 07]: 2-D preprocessing of the X-ray projection images, high-pass filtering in frequency domain of the X-ray projection images, back-projection and 3-D post-processing. Each projection image is processed instantaneously when it is transferred from the acquisition device over the network or, alternatively, when it is loaded from the hard disk. The back-projection is the computationally most expensive step and typically accounts for more than 70% of the overall execution time [Heig 07]. For each projection image and for each discrete volume element (voxel), the intersection of the corresponding X-ray beam with the detector is computed and the respective detector intensity is accumulated to the current voxel.

Figure 3.1 illustrates the processing steps in the order of occurrence. A more detailed discussion of algorithms used in reconstruction systems has already been presented in Chapter 2 or can alternatively be found in [Wies 00] and [Zell 05].

3.1.2 Target Hardware Platforms

Due to the immense processing requirements of any reconstruction system, acceleration with special hardware is mandatory in order to meet the requirements of today's medical workflow. Acceleration boards based upon FPGA technology have often been used in commercial reconstruction systems [Heig 07].

A combination of hardware using off-the-shelf technology may also be used for this task. Today, graphics accelerator boards, the CBEA, multi-core and multi-processor systems seem to be the most promising candidates. A significant advantage of these acceleration platforms over FPGA solutions is that their implementation requires much less development effort than FPGA-based solutions.

3.1.2.1 Multi-Core and Multi-Processor Systems

Nowadays, all relevant reconstruction systems are based upon this type of hardware. These systems are considered as the basic building block in every reconstruction system. The control flow of any reconstruction algorithm and some parts of it are often implemented on these processors. However, the processing power is still insufficient to achieve the reconstruction speed that is required in interventional environments. In addition, the computationally most expensive tasks must therefore be accelerated using special hardware architectures.

3.1.2.2   Cell Broadband Engine Architecture

The CBEA [Pham 05] introduced by IBM, Toshiba, and Sony is a special type of a multi-core processing system consisting of a PowerPC Processor Element (PPE) together with eight Synergistic Processor Elements (SPEs) offering a theoretical performance of 204.8 Gflops^2 (3.2 GHz, 8 SPEs, 4 floating point multiply-add operations per clock cycle) on a single chip. The processor is still completely programmable using high level languages such as C and C++.

The major challenge of porting an algorithm to the CBEA is to exploit the parallelism that it exhibits. The PPE, which is compliant with the 64-bit Power architecture, is dedicated to host a Linux operating system and manages the SPEs as resources for computationally intensive tasks. The SPEs support 128 bit vector instructions to execute the same operations simultaneously on multiple data elements (SIMD). In case of single precision floating point values (4 byte each) four operations can be executed in parallel. The SPEs are highly optimized for running compute-intensive code. They have only a small memory each (local store, 256 KB) and are connected to each other and to the main memory via a fast bus system, the Element Interconnect Bus (EIB). The data transfer between SPEs and main memory is not done automatically as is the case for conventional processor architectures, but is under complete control of the programmer, who can thus optimize data flow without any side effects of caching policies.

A more detailed overview of the CBEA is given in Section 4.1.

3.1.2.3   Common Unified Device Architecture

In comparison to the nine-way coherent CBEA, modern GPUs offer even more parallelism by their SIMD design paradigm. The Nvidia Tesla C1060 computing processor, for example, uses 240 Stream Processors in parallel offering a theoretical performance of 933 Gflops^2(240 stream processors, 1.296 GHz, one multiply-add operation and one multiply operation per clock cycle per Stream Processor).

Recently, Nvidia has provided a fundamentally new, and easy-to-use computing architecture for solving complex computational problems on the GPU. It is called the Common Unified Device Architecture (CUDA). It allows to implement graphics-accelerated applications using the C-programming language with a few CUDA-specific extensions.

The programs, which are executed on the graphics device, are called kernels. A graphics context must be initialized and bound to a thread running on the host system. The execution of the kernels must be initiated from this thread, which must be addressed in the design of the software architecture.

A more detailed overview of CUDA is presented in Section 6.1.

---

^{2} 1 Gflops = 1 Giga floating-point operations per second = 10^9 floating-point operations per second

3.2 Reconstruction System Design

Throughout the discussion of our reconstruction system design we suppose that the whole system is primarily based upon a general-purpose computing platform either as a single-core or multi-core system. This system may be extended by several hardware accelerators either on-chip or as an accelerator board. For this reason, the design must allow the acceleration by specific hardware architectures at each part of the algorithm. It is also required that several different hardware architectures can be used for different processing steps.

3.2.1 Reconstruction Pipeline

As can be seen in Figure 3.1 the overall computation of the reconstruction system involves performing calculations on a set of 2-D projection images, where the calculations can be viewed in terms of the projections flowing through a sequence of stages. We use the pipeline design pattern [Matt 05] to map the blocks (stages) of Figure 3.1 onto entities working together in order to form a powerful software framework which is both, reusable, as well as easy to maintain and to extend.

3.2.1.1 Pipeline Design Pattern

Software systems where ordered data passes through a series of processing tasks are ideally mapped to a pipeline architecture [Matt 05]. This is especially true for any CT reconstruction system where hundreds of X-ray projection images have to be processed in several filtering steps and are then back-projected into the resulting volume dataset. The pipeline pattern should be applied to build configurable data-flow pipelines. In our design we use a combination of the pipeline patterns that are described in [Posn 96, Verm 95]. In the following we review the pipeline design pattern in the context of a reconstruction system.

From the software engineering point of view, the pipeline design pattern provides the following benefits for the reconstruction system architecture:

- It allows to decouple the compositional structure of the processing tasks in a specific algorithm from the implementation that computes the respective tasks.

- It is possible to set up the pipeline in a type-safe and pluggable manner. Type-safe means that the type of data that is sent through the different pipeline stages can be defined and enforced statically by the compiler.

- The pipeline can be both configured and reconfigured dynamically and independently from reusable components.

Depending on the used reconstruction algorithm, the order of both control and data messages that are sent through the pipeline stages must often be preserved. This is easy to realize using the pipeline approach, because the pipeline design pattern depends upon the flow of data between stages.

3.2.1.2   Concurrency

Within the pipeline design pattern, the concurrent execution of the different stages is possible using a multi-threaded design approach. This allows us to compute the different parts of the reconstruction algorithm in parallel. The following factors affect the performance of reconstruction systems that are based upon this pattern:

- The slowest pipeline stage will determine the aggregate reconstruction speed.

- Communication overhead can affect the performance of the application, especially when only few computations are executed in a pipeline stage. In a reconstruction system, the granularity of the data flow between pipeline stages can be considered to be large, because most often projection images will flow through the pipeline as a whole. On shared-memory architectures, the number of computations that are performed on the projection images is high in comparison to the communication overhead.

- The amount of concurrency in the pipeline is limited by the number of pipeline stages and a larger number of pipeline stages is preferable. In a reconstruction system this number depends upon the reconstruction algorithm and is therefore limited considering a pipeline flow with a granularity of projection images.

- The time required to fill and drain the pipeline should be small compared to the overall run-time. Since reconstruction systems process a large amount of projections, this point can be ignored in this context.

Nonetheless, for a reconstruction system, the amount of concurrency offered by the pipeline pattern is by far insufficient. We therefore consider the pipeline architecture only as the basic building block of the overall reconstruction system architecture that structures and simplifies its implementation and enables basic concurrent processing. As will be described in Section 3.2.2, the actual strength of the pipeline design comes into play when we combine this pattern with the master/worker pattern for selected pipeline stages in order to make use of special accelerator hardware.

3.2.2   Parallelization Strategy

As was outlined in the previous section, the pipeline design pattern is able to act as the basic building block of a reconstruction system. In order to achieve the reconstruction speed necessary for the typical medical workflow, the level of concurrency in the pipeline design is still not sufficient and flexible enough. Therefore, the software architecture of a reconstruction system has to be extended by including other possibilities of achieving concurrency.

In this section we show how the gap can ideally be filled when combining the master/worker [Matt 05] design pattern with the pipeline design pattern.

3.2.2.1   Master/Worker Design Pattern

The master/worker design pattern is particularly useful for embarrassingly parallel problems that can be faced by a task parallelization approach [Matt 05]. The most computationally expensive task in a reconstruction system, the back-projection, is of such type. The master/worker approach is also applicable to a variety of parallel algorithm structures and it is possible to use it as a paradigm for hardware accelerated algorithm design on many different architectures. In the following we review the master/worker design pattern in the context of a reconstruction system.

The master divides the problem into tasks – in the following denoted as work instruction blocks (WIBs) – and sends them to its workers for processing. For example, the back-projection computation can be partitioned into several WIBs, each corresponding to a small sub-volume. Then, each worker processes in a loop one WIB after the other and sends the respective results back to the master. When the master received all WIBs corresponding to a specific task, the processing of that task is finished.

A parallelization strategy based upon the master/worker pattern has the following characteristics:

- Static and dynamic load balancing strategies can be applied for the distribution of the tasks to the workers. Both strategies are easy to realize. In Section 3.2.2.3 we will see that this is particularly important for hardware abstraction in our design.

- Master/worker algorithms have good scalability as long as the number of WIBs significantly exceeds the number of workers.

- The processing time of a task must be significantly higher than the necessary communication overhead to distribute it to a worker and back to the master.

The last two characteristics can easily be enforced in the considered medical imaging applications. For performance reasons all worker processes should be created when the pipeline is initialized. This saves the overhead resulting from frequent creation and termination of worker processes.

3.2.2.2 Combination with the Pipeline Design Pattern

From a macroscopic point of view, our software architecture consists of a pipeline structure. In order to overcome the limited flexibility and concurrency in the pipeline design pattern (see Section 3.2.1.2), further refinement of the pipeline stages is necessary. We propose a software design of the reconstruction system that allows a hierarchical composition of the pipeline and the master/worker design patterns. This allows to integrate a master and a configurable number of workers in a pipeline stage. In the context of our reconstruction task we have found that in the majority of cases it is sufficient to have only a hierarchy depth of one, which means that it must only be possible to integrate master/worker processing in a pipeline stage. Especially in multi GPU scenarios it is, however, a useful extension if pipelines can be nested in a specific worker. This procedure totally closes the gap of limited support for flexibility and concurrency in the pipeline pattern.

A centralized approach with only one master process can easily become a bottleneck when the master is not fast enough to keep all of its workers busy. It also prohibits an optimal usage of the acceleration hardware because its processing power still has to be assigned or partitioned statically to specific pipeline stages. For this reason, we extend our design such that it allows to share processing elements between several master/worker pipeline stages (see Section 3.2.3.1).

3.2.2.3   Hardware Abstraction

The combined pipeline and master/worker design paradigm can be used to parallelize most parts of a specific reconstruction algorithm and it is not tied to any particular hardware. The approach can be used for everything from clusters to shared-memory architectures. It can thus act as a hardware abstraction layer in the reconstruction system.

The basic functionality and communication mechanisms of the master/worker pattern have to be implemented only once for each supported hardware architecture, and different load balancing strategies can be integrated in its communication abstraction. This is necessary because for a specific hardware architecture, a certain load balancing strategy may be better than another one. For example, using a multi GPU platform and CUDA, the sharing of resources in device memory among a task-group can require static load balancing. In contrast to this, the CBEA always performs best with a dynamic load balancing approach, since no resources are shared in local store among task-groups.

In reconstruction systems, several hardware components may be used for the acceleration of different parts of the reconstruction algorithm. The combination of the pipeline and master/worker pattern has enough flexibility to support such heterogeneous systems allowing the usage of different acceleration hardware solutions in each pipeline stage. A specific part of the reconstruction algorithm may be mapped to the best suited acceleration hardware independently of the processing order. For example, multi-core systems may be used in between GPU-accelerated parts of the algorithm.

In combination with the factory design pattern [Alex 01, Gamm 94], most parts of the overall reconstruction algorithm can be expressed independently from the used acceleration hardware. This allows for a portable and flexible algorithm design that reuses the common parts and even enables the respective architecture execution configuration of the pipeline stages to be changed dynamically at run-time.

3.2.3   Resource Management

Another important aspect in the design of a reconstruction system is the resource management. We distinguish the relevant resources of the considered target hardware platforms into two classes: processing elements and data buffers. In the following we show how a sophisticated resource management can easily be integrated in the reconstruction system design for both processing elements and data buffers.

3.2.3.1   Processing Elements

As was outlined in Section 3.2.2.2, processing elements have to be statically assigned to special master/worker pipeline stages, which prohibits an optimal usage of the acceleration hardware. For this reason we want to share processing elements between several master/worker pipeline stages.

This is achieved by extending the single master methodology to support multiple masters, each of them living in a different pipeline stage, but still using the same group of workers. In this respect, the design is enhanced by an improved scalability and also by a reduction of the limitation that the slowest pipeline stage determines the aggregate reconstruction speed. Load is now automatically balanced between pipeline stages with master/worker processing capability that are using the same group of workers. Only this extension enables an optimal usage of the considered hardware architectures:

- In multi-processor and multi-core systems, thread switching overhead can be reduced by controlling the overall number of used threads.

- With regard to the CBEA, resource usage of the processing elements is especially improved by sharing the SPEs between pipeline stages. It is therefore necessary to technically compile each worker side of the shared pipeline stages into one associated SPE program. This may result in too large SPE program binaries which do not fit into the local store any more.

- In CUDA development, the considered design allows to share a single graphics context and thus GPU device resources among different pipeline stages, which avoids expensive data transfers between device and host memory.

3.2.3.2 Data Buffers

In a reconstruction system, resource management must also be addressed for data buffers, because the allocation of memory for all buffers is not always feasible. For example, the reconstruction of a typical medical dataset in C-arm CT requires up to three GB to store the reconstruction volume together with all projections. It is therefore necessary to allocate only a limited number of data buffers. That means that only a few projection images and the reconstruction volume may be used during reconstruction. In order to avoid the frequent allocation and deallocation of memory, which is an expensive operation, we reuse projection and volume buffers after they have been processed. This can be achieved by using the object pool pattern [Gran 98].

By introducing this design paradigm, data buffers can be acquired from the pool and released to the pool in any pipeline stage. For example, the projection buffers can be acquired in the first stage of the pipeline and released in the back-projection stage after processing. In order to support the multi-threaded software framework, the object pool can be based upon a shared queue object [Matt 05]. The pool will block any pop requests when no more data buffers are available and unblocks the respective request immediately as soon as a data buffer has been released to the pool.

3.3 Implementation

We implemented the discussed design approach in our RTK software framework. In the following we present the basic building blocks of our implementation. We abstract from all details that are not relevant to understand the basic structure of our implementation.

3.3.1   Structure

The UML class diagram in Figure 3.2 illustrates the inheritance hierarchy of our design approach.

3.3.2   Participants

All entities live in the *rtk* namespace which we do not qualify in the following for enhanced readability.

- **InputSide** defines the input interface of a pipeline stage for data items and control information.

- **OutputSide** defines the output interface of a pipeline stage for data items and control information.

- **Stage** combines an InputSide with an OutputSide to create an interior pipeline stage.

- **SourceStage** is the first pipeline stage in a pipeline. The source stage creates its input data items for its own in a separate thread of control and provides a mechanism for the application to start the execution of the pipeline.

- **SinkStage** is the last pipeline stage in a pipeline. It provides a mechanism for the application to wait for a result and to get it from the pipeline.

- **Port** manages the connection of two stages and provides the mechanism for output. The port concept enables the dynamic composition of two pipeline stages with active and passive read or write semantics [Verm 95] at run-time and without a complex class hierarchy.

- **NestedPort** manages the connection of two stages with active write and passive read semantics [Verm 95] in that order. The stages connected by this mechanism are sharing the same thread of execution.

- **ThreadedPort** manages the connection of two stages with active write and active read semantics [Verm 95] in that order. The stages connected by this mechanism will run in different threads of execution.

- **MasterStage** is the pipeline stage that is responsible for partitioning the processing into WIBs (scattering) and to respond to processed WIBs (gathering). The communication with its corresponding WorkerStage is done by a concrete Master. The MasterStage must therefore register at a concrete Master in order to use its communication abstraction and the processing elements that are managed by the corresponding Master.

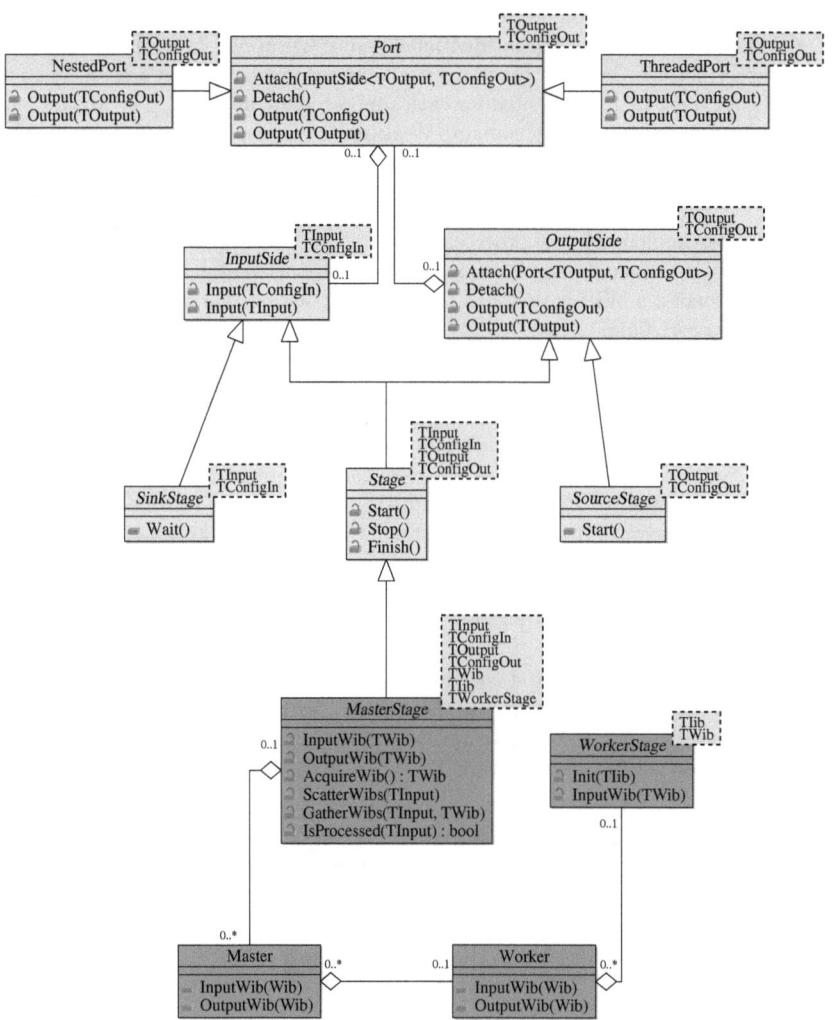

Figure 3.2: UML class diagram of the inheritance hierarchy of our design approach. The classes used to implement the pipeline pattern are shown in light gray. The combination with the master/worker pattern is illustrated by the added classes in dark gray.

- **WorkerStage** does the processing of a WIB for a corresponding MasterStage. All communication with the corresponding MasterStage is taken over by the corresponding concrete Master that controls this stage and the respective Worker.

- **Master** provides the basic functionality for the application of the master/-worker pattern. While it functions as the hardware abstraction layer a concrete Master must be implemented for each supported architecture. The Master also creates the corresponding concrete Workers for the respective architecture. The Master allows one or more MasterStages to connect to it and also initiates the creation of the corresponding WorkerStages.

- **Worker** implements the processing node of the corresponding Master. A concrete Worker must be implemented for each supported architecture. The actual processing of a WIB is switched to the corresponding WorkerStage which shall do the processing.

3.3.3   Sample Code and Usage

The following code samples illustrate how the CT reconstruction system from Section 3.1.1 could be implemented in C++. We concentrate on the implementation of this application using the RTK framework rather than going into the implementation details of the framework itself. As an example we assume that we want to accelerate the filtering step of the application using a general purpose multi-core platform and the preprocessing and back-projection shall be accelerated using two CUDA-enabled graphics cards. We intentionally skipped the postprocessing step in order to shorten the sample implementations.

The creation of the concrete stages that build up the pipeline is done by the factory class *PcCudaFactory* that implements the abstract factory providing the interface to the used methods. We refer to [Gamm 94] and [Alex 01] for more details about the factory and abstract factory pattern.

```cpp
// Param is the type that configures the stages
// Proj is the type for X-ray projection images
// Vol is the type of the reconstruction volume

// type of the filter pipeline stages
typedef Stage<Proj,Param,Proj,Param> FltStage;

// type of the back-projection pipeline stage
typedef Stage<Proj,Param,Vol,Param> BpStage;

class PcCudaFactory : public Factory {
public:
    // Default Constructor
    inline PcCudaFactory() :
        // use eight processing threads
        // on the multi-core architecture
        masterPc_ (8),
```

```
        // use two GPUs with CUDA
        masterCuda_ (2) {}
    // Creates the preprocessing stage with
    // hardware acceleration using CUDA
    inline FltStage* CreatePrepStage() {
        return new PrepMasterCuda(masterCuda_ );
    }
    // Creates the filtering stage with
    // acceleration using multi-core systems
    inline FltStage* CreateFltStage() {
        return new FltMasterPc(masterPc_ );
    }
    // Creates the back-projection stage with
    // hardware acceleration using CUDA
    inline BpStage* CreateBpStage() {
        return new BpMasterCuda(masterCuda_ );
    }
private:
    MasterPc    masterPc_ ;
    MasterCuda masterCuda_ ;
};
```

The preprocessing and back-projection pipeline stage share the same master, which also enables to share the two CUDA-enabled GPUs for their processing. The classes *PrepMasterCuda*, *FilterMasterPc* and *BpMasterCuda* implement the respective algorithms in an accelerated version using the mentioned hardware platforms. For the sake of this example we give a sketch of the back-projection implementation using the two CUDA-enabled GPUs. We have to implement two classes - the master pipeline stage *BpMasterCuda* and the corresponding worker stage *BpWorkerCuda*:

```
// Iib is the type of a init instruction block
// Wib is the type of a work instruction block

class BpWorkerCuda :
        public WorkerStage<Proj, Iib, Wib> {
private:
    virtual void Init(const Iib& iib) {
        bp_init_cuda(iib);
    }
    virtual void InputWib(const Iib& iib,
                                Wib& wib) {
        bp_process_cuda(iib, wib);
    }
};

class BpMasterCuda : public MasterStage<Proj,
        Param, Vol, Param, Iib, Wib, BpWorkerCuda> {
private:
    virtual void Configure(
```

```
                        const Param& config) {
        currentVolume_ = CreateVolume(config);
    }
    virtual void Finish() {
        Output(*currentVolume_);
        currentVolume_ = 0;
    }
    virtual void ScatterWibs(Proj& proj) {
        // process all sub-volumes
        for (int i=0; i<2; ++i) {
            // Get a new wib
            Wib& wib = AcquireWib(proj);
            // Initialize wib for sub-volume
            InitWib(wib, i);
            // Send wib to worker
            OutputWib(wib);
        }
    }
    virtual void GatherWibs(Proj& proj,
                            Wib& wib) {
        // handle processed wib
        if (IsProcessed(proj))
            ReleaseInput(proj);
    }
    // Pointer to the reconstruction volume
    Vol* currentVolume_;
};
```

Within the main function of the application we need to construct a source stage, which loads the projection images and a sink stage that stores the volume. For each processing step of the reconstruction pipeline we further construct the MasterStage using the factory.

```
// construct factory, source and sink
PcCudaFactory factory;
SourceStage<Proj, Param> source;
SinkStage<Vol, Param> sink;

// construct the master stages
// for preprocessing
FltStage* prep = factory.CreatePrepStage();
// for filtering
FltStage* flt = factory.CreateFltStage();
// and for back-projection
BpStage* bp = factory.CreateBpStage();
```

Now it is just a matter of building up the pipeline.

```
// type of the used port class
// that has a separate thread of execution
typedef ThreadedPort<Proj, Param> Threaded;
// that shares the thread of execution
```

```
typedef NestedPort<Vol, Param> Nested;

// connect pipeline stages
Pipeline :: Connect(&source, prep, new Threaded ());
Pipeline :: Connect(prep, flt, new Threaded ());
Pipeline :: Connect(flt, bp, new Threaded ());
Pipeline :: Connect(bp, &sink, new Nested ());

// start pipeline and wait for the result
source . Start ();
sink . Wait ();
```

With a different implementation of the Factory class the pipeline can be easily configured to use different hardware acceleration platforms for each processing steps without changing most parts of the implementation.

3.4 Summary

We have presented both the design and implementation of a software architecture that is well suited to implement and accelerate the computationally intensive task of 3-D reconstruction in medical imaging. Software engineering techniques play an important role in the overall design and can improve the efficiency, flexibility and portability of the whole reconstruction system.

In this regard, we have shown that the underlying software architecture can be mapped to a design approach that combines the pipeline design pattern with the master/worker design pattern. We have illustrated how the design can act as a hardware abstraction layer to different acceleration architectures. Finally, we have demonstrated that it even enables the combination of several acceleration hardware platforms for different parts of the algorithm in a heterogeneous system.

Chapter 4

Cell Broadband Engine Architecture

Long before other microprocessor chip vendors developed wide spread multi-core processors Sony Computer Entertainment, Toshiba, and IBM formed an allegiance (commonly known as STI-allegiance) to build a highly multi-core processor that can overcome the problems of traditional microprocessor technology. The outcome was the *Cell Broadband Engine Architecture* [Cell06, Pham05] which mainly targets three different market shares. The first major commercial application of the Cell processor was Sony's activity to penetrate the gaming market with the Cell-based PlayStation 3 video game console. Further application domains of the Cell processor are in the multimedia industry and in the high performance computing community. For example, IBM's latest supercomputer, the IBM Roadrunner, is a hybrid system consisting of General Purpose CISC Opteron processors as well as PowerXCell 8i Cell processors. In June 2008 this supercomputer ranked first in the TOP500 list[1], which maintains the list of the world's most powerful supercomputers, reaching record-breaking one Petaflop – a quadrillion floating-point operations per second – of compute power using the standard Linpack benchmark.

The Cell processor could be an ideal candidate to accelerate cone-beam CT image reconstruction, which is one of the most compute intensive applications in the medical industry. The programming methodology of the CBEA, however, pose a major challenge to software developers who wish to make the most of this horsepower, demanding careful hand-tuning of programs to extract maximal performance from this processor.

In the following we evaluate the applicability and suitability of the Cell processor in the context of cone-beam CT reconstruction. In the next section we cover the architecture of the CBEA. Then we develop a highly optimized CBEA-based implementation of the FDK method (Section 4.2) and present the achieved results (Section 4.3). The main contributions of this chapter have been presented at the SPIE Medical Imaging Conference 2007 [Sche07c].

4.1 Architecture

The CBEA is a general-purpose multi-core processor consisting of a Power Processor Element (PPE) together with eight Synergistic Processor Elements (SPEs) offering a

---

[1]http://www.top500.org

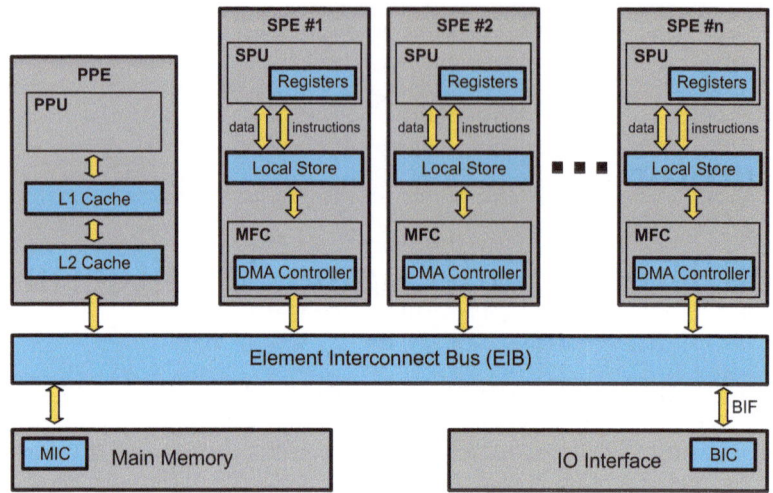

Figure 4.1: Architecture of the Cell processor.

theoretical performance of 204.8 Gflops (3.2 GHz, 8 SPEs, 4 floating-point multiply and add per clock cycle) on a single chip. Figure 4.1 gives an overview of the architecture of the Cell processor. The processor is still completely programmable using high level languages such as C and C++. The major challenge of porting an algorithm to the CBEA is to exploit the parallelism that it exhibits. The PPE, which is compliant with the 64-bit Power architecture, is dedicated to host a Linux operating system and manages the SPEs as resources for computationally intensive tasks. The SPEs support 128 bit vector instructions to execute the same operations simultaneously on multiple data elements (SIMD: Single Instruction Multiple Data) [Oh 06]. In case of single precision floating-point values (4 bytes each) four operations can be executed at the same time. The SPEs are highly optimized for running compute-intensive code. They have only a small memory each (Local Store, 256 KB) and are connected to each other and to the main memory via a fast bus system, the Element Interconnect Bus (EIB). The data transfer between SPEs and main memory is not done automatically as is the case for conventional processor architectures, but is under complete control of the programmer, who can thus optimize data flow without any side effects of cache replacement strategies.

In the following sections we give a detailed overview of the main components of the CBEA.

4.1.1   The Power Processor Element

The PPE is a two-way multithreaded core which is compliant with the 64-bit Power Architecture. It works with conventional operating systems, but currently only the Linux operating system is supported. The Power Processor Unit (PPU) within the PPE is a dual-issue, in-order processor. Up to two instructions can be issued at the same time as long as they do not utilize the same execution unit. In order to optimize the use of instruction issue slots, two instructions from two different threads are interleaved. The processor appears to the operating system as two independent processors although the computational resources are shared between them.

The PPE contains a 32 KB instruction cache and a cache hierarchy consisting of a 32 KB first-level cache and a 512 KB second-level cache for accesses to main memory. The size of a cache line is 128 bytes. The PPU further supports the Vector/SIMD Multimedia Extension of the PowerPC architecture via its AltiVec unit which is fully pipelined for single precision floating-point. Double-precision floating-point vectors are not supported. While each PPU can complete two floating-point operations per clock cycle using a scalar-fused multiply-add instruction, the theoretical peak performance of the PPE is capable of 6.4 Gflops in double-precision at 3.2 GHz. In single precision the peak performance translates even to 25.6 Gflops using a vector-fused multiply-add instruction of eight floating-point operations each.

Most of the time, however, the PPE acts only as the controller for up to eight SPEs, which are used to handle most of the computational workload.

4.1.2 The Synergistic Processor Elements

The SPEs are optimized for compute intensive code. Each SPE is composed of a Synergistic Processor Unit (SPU), and a Memory Flow Controller (MFC). The SPU is a RISC[2] processor with 128-bit SIMD organization for single and double precision instructions. Its instruction-set architecture was designed to provide immense performance capability for compute-intensive applications. It contains a large register file having 128 entries and it can either operate on sixteen 8-bit integers, eight 16-bit integers, four 32-bit integers, or four single precision floating-point numbers in a single clock cycle, as well as a memory operation. Thus, two instructions can be issued per cycle, one on the even pipeline which performs fixed and floating-point arithmetics and one on the odd pipeline which executes load, store and byte permutation operations. Both instruction scheduling and branch prediction is done in a static way, which means that the ordering and the addresses of instructions decide whether they are executed as single- or dual-issue. At 3.2 GHz, each SPE thus gives a theoretical 25.6 Gflops of single precision floating-point performance.

In Figure 4.1 it can be seen that the SPU cannot directly access the system's main memory. Instead the Local Store (LS) has to be used. It contains a 256 KB embedded SRAM for both the program code and the data used during processing. The Local Store is very different from a conventional CPU cache since it is neither transparent to software nor does it contain hardware structures that predict which data to load. This requires to explicitly use the MFC to initiate DMA (Direct Memory Access) commands and to transfer data between local memory and system main memory. Multiple memory transfers may be active at the same time while the SPU processes data from the Local Store. In this way memory latencies can be effectively hidden and the full memory access bandwidth can be utilized.

Compared to a modern personal computer, the SPEs provide relatively high overall floating-point performance for an application. However, the software programming

---

[2] Reduced instruction set computer (RISC)

approach of the CBEA makes it very difficult to implement and to optimize software because of the limited size of the Local Store, the necessity to implement data transfers to and from the Local Store manually, and the usage of vector instructions. This poses a major challenge to software developers who wish to efficiently use the offered compute capability, demanding careful hand-tuning of programs in order to extract maximal performance from this processor. Rudimentary compiler support at least for automatic vectorization has been available but delivered unsatisfying results.

On the other hand, due to the flexible nature of the Cell, there are several programming approaches possible in order to utilize its resources, not limited to just different computing paradigms.

4.1.3   The Element Interconnect Bus

The EIB is a data transfer bus internal to the Cell processor. It connects the PPE and the SPEs with the memory controller, and the bus interface controller. It presently consists of four circular rings connecting all devices in the same order. Data transfer on these rings is unidirectional, two of the rings transfer clockwise and the other one goes counterclockwise. The EIB can sustain a data rate of over 200 GB/s where each port has a bandwidth of 25.6 GB/s. The bandwidth for accessing main memory is also 25.6 GB/s.

It is required to adapt the parallel implementation of an algorithm to the physical structure of the EIB. Bottlenecks can arise if multiple devices access a single port, e.g. the MIC, and overlaps of data transfers of the rings can limit the overall bandwidth. The latencies for data transfers can, however, be effectively hidden for compute intensive tasks. For workloads caused by such applications the performance of the EIB is sufficient even if its physical structure is not considered.

4.2   Feldkamp Algorithm

We mapped the processing chain of the FDK method to the pipeline architecture of the RTK framework by executing the filtering and back-projection on dedicated stages, respectively, using a different thread of control for each stage. In order to utilize the processing elements of the Cell processor, we used the Master/Worker approach of the framework to dispatch the associated parallel processing of a stage to a configurable number of workers (SPEs or PPEs). In our implementation the PPE acts as the master which divides the processing of the considered stage into smaller tasks and assigns them to the available processing units (SPEs). This concept is flexible with respect to the number of SPEs that are available for the processing while others might be busy with other tasks like filtering or preprocessing data.

To minimize the control overhead we assign rather large tasks to the processing elements that further have to be divided into smaller tasks by the processing elements themselves. We take special care to hide any communication latencies via double buffering techniques during the dispatching and computation process. The only downside of our approach is that the mapping of the SPEs onto the stages is currently done statically. This means that we have to decide which SPEs shall be used for the filtering or back-projection stage before program execution. Our approach can be extended to reduce the number of utilized SPEs for each stage dynamically, if higher priority tasks are waiting to be dispatched in other pipeline stages.

An efficient implementation on the CBEA further requires to choose a proper parallelization strategy for each algorithm that can deal with the limited Local Store size.

4.2.1 Filtering

During the filtering we assign several projection rows to an SPE at the same time. The SPE can process simultaneously two rows by loading them into its Local Store, and performing the Fourier-based convolution after adding the required zero-padding. Fortunately, the Cell SDK provided a sufficiently efficient FFT implementation for the SPEs as open source, which is used in our implementation. Finally, communication latencies are effectively hidden via double buffering techniques.

4.2.2 Back-Projection

Although the RTK framework already removes much of the complexity of using the Cell SDK, a lot of code transformations are necessary in order to adapt the back-projection code to the Cell architecture. Despite of the code optimizations of the innermost back-projection loop, a parallelization strategy must be developed which is able to handle the limited size of the Local Store in the SPEs. In this regard a parallel implementation of the back-projection algorithm requires to divide the problem into smaller and independent tasks that can be assigned to the available processing units.

4.2.2.1 Problem Partitioning

Two critical resources have to be considered when creating tasks for an SPE: the small amount of local memory and the limited communication bandwidth between main memory and the SPEs. One basic back-projection task takes a small sub-volume and the associated projection data as input. The updated sub-volume data is written back to main memory after computation. It must further be guaranteed that different SPEs do not work on the same sub-volumes.

Sub-Volume Shape. The projection data which a sub-volume depends on is given by the convex hull of the sub-volume corner points projected onto the image plane (see Figure 4.2). This region will be referred to as the *projection shadow* of the sub-volume. In order to simplify the handling of the projection shadows we use a rectangular bounding box around its convex hull, which is parallel to the coordinate axes of the detector.

While the memory requirements for sub-volume data are determined by its dimensions only, the size of the projection shadow depends on a variety of parameters of the acquisition geometry, the discretization (voxel and pixel size), and the shape of the sub-volume, together with the position of the sub-volume within the volume of interest (VOI). In principle the following analysis of the sub-volume shape must be done for each dataset separately. The acquisition geometry, however, can be expected to be constant for a certain device even though different calibration results and scan protocols might lead to slight variations.

In the following we investigate an optimal sub-volume shape for a typical dataset of a state-of-the-art C-arm device (see Appendix B.2). The dataset is reconstructed using a volume which contains the whole VOI and which consists of 512^3 voxels. The voxel size is 0.46 mm in each dimension. Using larger voxel sizes will result in significantly bigger projection shadows. It is then required either to use smaller sub-volumes or to downsample the projection images.

The sub-volume shape was optimized by simulating the maximum projection shadow size and the overall amount of projection data that has to be transferred for the mentioned acquisition geometry and discretization. Table 4.1 summarizes the achieved results. The required Local Store memory is simply the sum of the sub-volume size and the maximal shadow. However, if double buffering (see Section 4.2.2.2) and bilinear interpolation (see Section 4.2.2.3) are used, the memory requirements increase by a factor of two for the sub-volume and even by a factor of four for the projection shadow.

While these optimization techniques are essential in order to achieve good performance we analyze the memory requirements such that the optimizations can be enabled. It can be seen that a suitable sub-volume shape is large in x- and y-direction, but small in z-direction. This can be intuitively explained by the fact that the main direction of projection rays is roughly parallel to the x-y-plane and therefore each pixel of the projection shadow is required more often in the computation for that sub-volume.

We decided for a sub-volume size of $32 \times 32 \times 8$ voxels, which is a good trade-off between memory requirements and overall amount of data transfer. This configuration has the further advantage that the memory size in x-direction of the sub-volume is a multiple of 128 bytes which results in an optimal memory transfer bandwidth between main memory and SPEs even if the complete volume is stored in row major memory format.

Task Assignment. Due to the limited Local Store size it is not possible to load the required projection shadows for all projections into the Local Store at the same time. Therefore, the required projection shadows have to be streamed to the SPEs while the data for one sub-volume is kept in Local Store memory.

The total number of sub-volumes N_S, which have to be processed for the dataset under consideration using the considered sub-volume dimensions, can be calculated by

$$N_S = \frac{512 \times 512 \times 512}{32 \times 32 \times 8} = 16384. \tag{4.1}$$

A very easy and efficient parallelization strategy could process the back-projection for one sub-volume and for all projection images of the dataset in one task. This would only require the creation of 16384 tasks (Equation 4.1) in order to reconstruct the complete dataset. Such a workload can be easily handled in a Master/Worker approach by the PPE as the master. This approach, however, has two obvious drawbacks. First, an enormous amount of main memory would be required in order to keep all projection images in main memory. For example, the reconstruction of the

Sub-Volume Dimensions [px]	Sub-Volume Size [KB]	Maximal Shadow [KB]	Required LS-Memory [KB]	Projection Data Transfer [GB]
16 x 16 x 4	4	7	36	226
16 x 16 x 8	8	10	56	185
16 x 16 x 12	12	13	76	172
16 x 16 x 16	**16**	**17**	**100**	**164**
24 x 24 x 4	9	12	66	146
24 x 24 x 8	18	16	100	115
24 x 24 x 12	27	20	134	105
24 x 24 x 16	**36**	**25**	**172**	**100**
24 x 24 x 20	45	29	206	97
24 x 24 x 24	54	34	244	95
32 x 32 x 4	16	17	100	106
32 x 32 x 8	**32**	**23**	**156**	**81**
32 x 32 x 12	48	28	208	73
32 x 32 x 16	64	34	264	68
32 x 32 x 20	80	39	316	66
32 x 32 x 24	96	45	372	65
32 x 32 x 28	112	51	428	63
32 x 32 x 32	128	56	480	62
48 x 48 x 4	**36**	**27**	**180**	**77**
48 x 48 x 8	72	33	276	56
48 x 48 x 12	108	39	372	49
48 x 48 x 16	144	46	472	45
64 x 64 x 16	256	72	800	33
64 x 64 x 24	384	89	1124	30
64 x 64 x 32	512	107	1452	28

Table 4.1: Memory requirements and amount of projection data transfer for different sub-volume sizes. Better configurations are written in bold letters.

considered dataset consisting of 543 projection images would require at least 2.4 GB of main memory only to save the projection images. Second, the back-projection processing can only start when all projection images are available and are loaded into main memory. An on-the-fly reconstruction would not be possible.

In order to enable an on-the-fly reconstruction with minimal main memory requirements a back-projection task may be reduced to the back-projection of a single projection image into only one sub-volume. Now both the sub-volumes and the corresponding projection shadows have to be streamed to the SPEs. This approach solves both problems mentioned above. However, using the Master/Worker approach to distribute the processing to the workers (SPEs), a lot more back-projection tasks have to be managed by the master (PPE):

$$N_S = \frac{512 \times 512 \times 512}{32 \times 32 \times 8} \times 543 = 8896512. \tag{4.2}$$

This may result in a back-projection performance that is limited by communication and synchronization issues. There are two possibilities to significantly reduce the computational effort for creating tasks on the PPE and the amount of communication required to transfer task information to the SPEs:

1. Multiple projection images can be combined to projection sequences. Very large projection sequence sizes, however, shall be avoided because more main memory has to be used to load a projection sequence and the on-the-fly reconstruction ability is reduced. Back-projection processing may not start until at least one complete projection sequence is loaded to main memory and the execution time of the back-projection processing increases by the time that is needed to process the last projection sequence. A projection sequence size of eight to 16 projections is a good compromise for the considered configuration. The number of projection buffers in main memory shall be at least twice as big as the size of the projection sequence in order to allow the processing of the following projection images in the previous stages while the current images are back-projected.

2. Another possibility to reduce the number of back-projection tasks is to combine several sub-volumes to a volume partition (see Figure 4.2). Then each worker (SPE) is responsible to further divide the volume partition into sub-volumes, which allows the worker to process all sub-volumes of that partition without further synchronization with its master.

The implementation of the algorithm uses the Master/Worker facilities of the RTK. In this regard the back-projection is implemented in a *MasterStage* on the PPE and in the corresponding *WorkerStages* on the SPEs. The master queues incoming projection images. As soon as a complete projection sequence is available it creates several back-projection tasks consisting of information about the volume partition and about the projection sequence. Each task is sent to an SPE in a work instruction block (WIB). Its contents are shown in Table 4.2. The RTK framework completely hides the CBEA specific implementation, which uses the hardware mailbox mechanism and DMA transfers to send and receive WIBs on the PPE and the

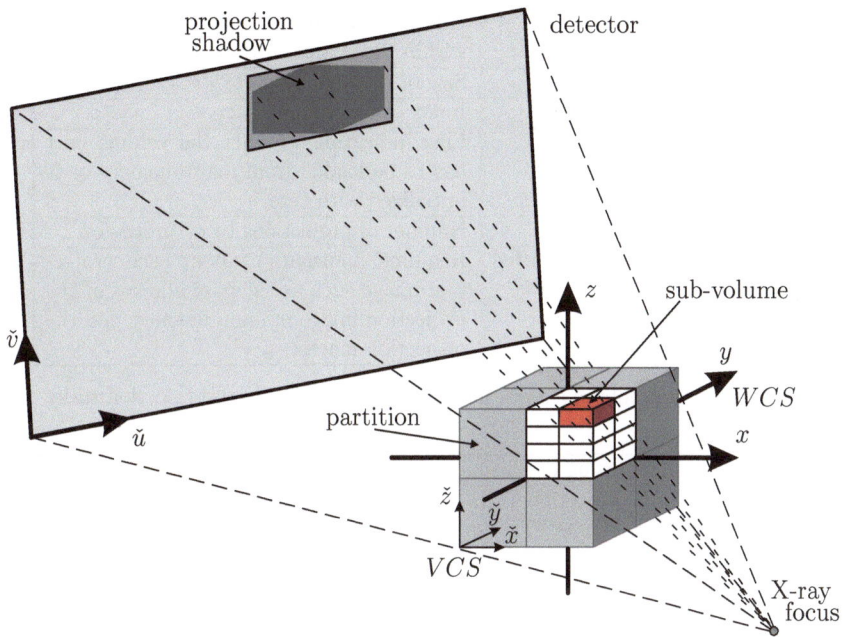

Figure 4.2: Perspective geometry of the cone-beam CT device (the $\check{v}$-axis and $\check{z}$-axis are not necessarily parallel) together with the parallelization strategy of our back-projection implementation using multi-core processors such as the CBEA (partitions are sent as tasks to the processing cores, and are then further subdivided into sub-volumes).

SPE. After the back-projection is finished, the reconstructed volume is handed over to the next *Stage* of the corresponding *Pipeline*. Algorithm 4 gives an overview of the subdivision scheme which is used to process the back-projection for one WIB on the SPE.

In order to avoid that the same sub-volume is processed by two different SPEs at the same time, we simply eliminate any possibility to process the same volume part by different SPEs. Therefore the master maintains a state variable for each volume part indicating if a WIB has already been sent to a worker but has not yet been processed. Each time the master creates a new WIB for a volume part it decides by this state variable if the WIB may be sent to a worker for processing or not. If the WIB currently cannot be sent to a worker it is put into the corresponding waiting queue for that partition in order to process it at a later time. After a WIB is processed, the corresponding waiting queue is checked for pending WIBs and they are assigned to a worker, if necessary.

The RTK framework provides a WIB queue for each worker and uses double buffering techniques to efficiently transfer the WIBs between master and workers. In order to exploit this mechanism in an optimal manner the number of independent

VolumePartOffset	Offset of the volume part to be processed within the complete volume
VolumePartSize	Size of the volume part
VolumePartIndex	Index of the volume part
VolumeIsInitialized	Flag indicating whether the volume part has to be loaded from main memory or is initialized with zero
Projections	Number of projections to be processed
ProjectionInfo[Projections]	Required information about each projection image such as the base address of the projection image in main memory and the projection matrix

Table 4.2: Contents of a work instruction block for a back-projection task.

Algorithm 4: Processing of a back-projection WIB.

Input: Back-projection WIB

1 **foreach** (*sub-volume V_s of the current partition*) **do**
2 $\quad$ Initiate DMA transfer to load sub-volume V_s;
3 $\quad$ Wait for DMA transfers of V_s;
4 $\quad$ **foreach** (*projection image $I_i, i \leq 0 < wib.Projections$*) **do**
5 $\quad\quad$ Initiate DMA transfer to load I_i;
6 $\quad\quad$ Wait for DMA transfers of I_i;
7 $\quad\quad$ Back-project(I_i, V_s);
8 $\quad$ **end**
9 $\quad$ Initiate DMA transfer to store sub-volume V_s;
10 $\quad$ Wait for DMA transfers of V_s;
11 **end**

WIBs, e.g. the number of volume parts, must be higher than the utilized number of SPEs. In order to keep 16 SPEs busy with work, it turns out that it is sufficient to divide the volume into 64 partitions. In this case four WIBs can be queued for each SPE.

Data Transfer Analysis. Because the total amount of projection data transfer D_P can hardly be expressed as an analytical expression, we simulated it by a separate program. The results are listed in Table 4.1. The projection data transfer for the considered dataset and the chosen sub-volume configuration thus accounts for memory transfers of 81 GB between SPEs and main memory.

Using our parallelization strategy the sub-volume data has to be transferred twice (once for reading and once for writing) for each back-projection task. In order to decrease the communication of volume data between main memory and the SPEs, several projection images can be combined to a single back-projection task for simul-

| Projection Sequence | Data Transfer | | |
Size	Volume [GB]	Projections [GB]	Total [GB]
1	543.0	81.0	624.0
2	271.5	81.0	352.5
4	135.8	81.0	216.8
8	67.9	81.0	148.9
16	33.9	81.0	114.9

Table 4.3: Main memory data transfer during back-projection processing of a dataset consisting of 512^3 voxels and using sub-volumes with a size of $32 \times 32 \times 8$

taneous processing, as it is already done to decrease the overall number of projection tasks. The overall amount of volume data transfer is thus given by

$$D_V = N_x \times N_y \times N_z \times 4Bytes \times 2 \times \frac{N_P}{N_{PS}}. \tag{4.3}$$

N_P denotes the total number of projection images and N_{PS} the size of a projection sequence. N_x, N_y, and N_z are the numbers of voxels of the volume in each dimension, respectively. Table 4.3 shows the total amount of data transfer for back-projection tasks using different projecion sequence sizes. It can be seen that at least eight projections should be combined into a single back-projection task.

4.2.2.2 Main Memory Access

In the previous section we developed a parallelization approach, which reduces the overall amount of data transfers while not being bottlenecked by communication latencies. In order to gain good memory access performance, however, data alignment, paging and locality of the data must be considered.

To further speed up access in main memory, we store the sub-volumes sequentially. So the complete volume is stored sub-volume by sub-volume, instead of line by line, plane by plane in main memory. In order to mitigate TLB-thrashing[3] we use huge pages of 16 MB size.

By applying the double buffering technique, where the computation uses one data buffer while the other one is transferred using a DMA command, we are able to hide data transfer times completely for the back-projection of high-resolution volumes. A drawback of the double buffering scheme is the required amount of Local Store memory for the additional projection and sub-volume buffers. In the last section, however, we showed a practical data partitioning scheme which allows to apply the double buffering technique during the reconstruction of a real medical CT dataset.

4.2.2.3 Code Optimization

For an efficient implementation of an algorithm on the SPEs one has to exploit their SIMD capabilities and enable a good instruction scheduling to the two pipelines of

---

[3] A translation lookaside buffer (TLB) is a CPU cache that memory management hardware uses to improve virtual address translation speed.

Interpolation mode	nearest neighbor		bilinear unoptimized		bilinear optimized	
SPE execution pipeline	even	odd	even	odd	even	odd
Address computation	14	1	17	1	15	1
Projection access	0	14	10	56	10	30
Voxel increment	3	2	3	2	3	2
Total	17	17	30	59	28	33

Table 4.4: Number of instructions required for the back-projection of a vector of voxels from one projection image.

each SPE. When looking at the back-projection for a single voxel from one projection image, one can identify the following three steps:

- Compute the projection coordinates and the address of the associated projection pixel.

- Read the value of that pixel using nearest neighbor or bilinear interpolation.

- Apply voxel-dependent distance weighting and increment the voxel value appropriately.

The first and the last step can be vectorized by performing the computations for multiple voxels in parallel. We choose to use vector instructions for neighboring voxels in x-direction, because each of the sub-volumes is stored in that order. The second step cannot be vectorized, because the required projection values will usually not be located in consecutive and aligned memory as required by a vector operation. Each SPE can issue simultaneously in each cycle (vector) instructions into two different pipelines. The even pipeline performs fixed and floating-point arithmetic while the odd pipeline executes only load, store, and byte permutation operations. By a proper scheduling of instructions, an optimal "cycles per instruction" (CPI) ratio of 0.5 can be achieved. Table 4.4 shows the numbers of instructions required for our algorithm with different interpolation modes on the two execution pipelines of the SPEs. While the address computation and voxel increment mainly require arithmetic instructions that are executed on the even pipeline, the projection data access is executed on the odd pipeline. We applied loop-unrolling techniques to the iteration over the voxels of a sub-volume in order to leverage efficient instruction scheduling and achieved code with a CPI ratio of 0.57 for the case of nearest neighbor interpolation.

Note the high number of instructions required for the data access. This is due to the fact that the SPEs cannot access basic data elements randomly in a vectorized way. Up to four instructions are required to load a single value: rotate the address into the preferred slot of a vector register, load the appropriate vector from memory, rotate the required element into the preferred slot, and finally shuffle it into the destination slot of the destination vector [Syne 05]. This is especially a problem for bilinear interpolation since, in this case, four projection pixels have to be accessed for each voxel update. This results in poor performance, if bilinear interpolation is implemented in a straightforward manner. We decreased the number of instructions required for the memory access during the back-projection by adapting the data layout of the loaded projection shadow before performing the actual back-projection. Therefore, we duplicated for each projection pixel the neighboring column pixel value into the same vector. This allows us to access two values with just one vector load instruction and therefore requires only two memory accesses per voxel. The data layout adaption can be performed at low computational cost because it can be vectorized efficiently. The drawback of this method is of course that it requires twice as much memory to store the projection shadow on the SPEs.

4.3 Results

The filtering and back-projection code was executed on a Blade server board based on the Cell architecture. Again the measurements were done using the datasets described in Appendix B.

In order to assess the performance of our implementation we used the "gettimeofday" function on the PPE. This ensures that all overhead during program execution (e.g., starting the SPE threads) are included in the measurements. In contrast, runtime measurements solely relying on the SPE decrementer (performance counter on SPE side) do only include the SPE program runtime, and a representative of all distinct SPE measurements has to be chosen. We perceived that measurements relying on the SPE decrementer lead to slightly reduced runtime (approximately 0.1 to 0.2 seconds below the runtime measured with "gettimeofday").

During our measurements we removed any outliers by taking only the best runtime out of five measurements, although runtime deviations of our experiments were only around 0.01 seconds. After the correctness of the implementation was verified, we performed the measurements without doing the I/O transfers for loading the projection images from the hard disk or over the network. This was necessary, in order to achieve runtime measurements that were not affected by I/O bandwidth limitations in our current Cell Blade evaluation system.

In a first step, we measured the performance of the filtering code and the back-projection code separately. Finally, we validated the performance of the overall pipeline execution (simultaneous, parallel execution of filtering and back-projection in a pipeline) for various partitioning configurations.

4.3.1 Filtering

The results of the filter execution using 1, 2, 3, 8, and 16 SPEs are shown in Table 4.5. The speed-up factor relative to the execution with only one SPE is also given, together with the numbers of projections that can be processed in one second (pps). Using all 16 SPEs filtering can be done in 0.49 seconds for Dataset (a) and in 1.02 seconds for Dataset (b). The FFT computations accounted for 86.71% of the total processing time for Dataset (a) and for 90.78% of the total processing time for Dataset (b). Data transfer time was negligible for Dataset (b), but consumed 1.11% of processing time for Dataset (a) and even increased approximately to 5% if all 16 SPEs are used for

Number of SPEs	1	2	3	8	16
Dataset (a), convolution length 2048					
Time [s]	5.84	2.97	1.99	0.82	0.49
Speed-up	1.00	1.97	2.93	7.09	11.80
pps	70.93	139.44	207.95	503.03	836.80
Dataset (b), convolution length 4096					
Time [s]	14.64	7.35	4.91	1.89	1.02
Speed-up	1.00	1.99	2.98	7.75	14.42
pps	37.09	73.84	110.62	287.50	534.96

Table 4.5: Performance results of Fourier-based filtering for the two considered datasets (convolution length is 2048 and 4096, respectively, due to zero-padding).

the computation. This is the reason why speed-up factors do not scale up linearly, especially not for the smaller dataset.

4.3.2   Back-Projection

We back-projected the cone-beam projections of the two datasets under consideration into a volume consisting of $512 \times 512 \times 512$ voxels. We chose 0.26^3 mm^3 for Dataset (a), and 0.31^3 mm^3 for Dataset (b) as the largest possible isotropic voxel size where still all voxels were inside the FOV (see Appendix B for more details).

In Table 4.6 we show the achieved results when executing only the back-projection using up to 16 SPEs of our dual Cell Blade for both datasets. The results have been measured using nearest neighbor and bilinear interpolation mode. Again, we give the speed-up factors relative to the execution with only one SPE and the number of projections that can be back-projected per second (pps). For convenience, we also calculated the number of 512×512 volume slices, that can be reconstructed in one second (frames per second, fps).

In nearest neighbor interpolation mode more than 30 projections can be reconstructed per second using only seven SPEs, which is sufficient for on-the-fly-reconstruction that is synchronized to the acquisition. Real-time imaging capability is also achieved in bilinear interpolation mode as soon as more than 12 SPEs are used for the back-projection.

The speed-up factor scales almost linearly, thus indicating that our back-projection implementation is not affected by memory bandwidth limitation. We could not observe communication latencies when profiling our code by instrumenting it with the SPE decrementer (performance counter on SPE side) either.

Right now, we considered only reconstruction volumes that are contained completely inside the FOV. When increasing the voxel size, parts of the cubic voxel volume will be outside the cylindrical FOV, and hence no meaningful values can be reconstructed in these regions any more. Our optimized implementation takes advantage of this by ignoring any voxels that lie outside the FOV.

In Figure 4.3 we show the achieved performance of FOV optimized reconstructions using Dataset (a) for volumes with an increased voxel size, such that only 78.26%,

Number of SPEs	1	6	7	**8**	14	15	**16**
Dataset (a), nearest neighbor interpolation							
Time [s]	93.13	15.71	13.50	**11.85**	6.89	6.47	**6.07**
Speed-up	1.00	5.93	6.90	**7.86**	13.51	14.40	**15.33**
pps	4.45	26.35	30.67	**34.94**	60.05	63.99	**68.16**
fps	5.50	32.58	37.94	**43.21**	74.26	79.14	**84.29**
Dataset (b), nearest neighbor interpolation							
Time [s]	122.34	20.53	17.64	**15.44**	8.97	8.39	**7.89**
Speed-up	1.00	5.96	6.94	**7.92**	13.65	14.58	**15.51**
pps	4.44	26.45	30.79	**35.17**	60.57	64.73	**68.85**
fps	4.18	24.94	29.03	**33.16**	57.11	61.03	**64.92**
Dataset (a), bilinear interpolation							
Time [s]	166.50	27.91	23.96	**20.99**	12.12	11.38	**10.68**
Speed-up	1.00	5.97	6.95	**7.93**	13.74	14.63	**15.60**
pps	2.49	14.83	17.28	**19.73**	34.16	36.38	**38.78**
fps	3.08	18.34	21.37	**24.40**	42.25	45.00	**47.96**
Dataset (b), bilinear interpolation							
Time [s]	220.37	36.88	31.65	**27.72**	16.02	14.95	**14.02**
Speed-up	1.00	5.97	6.96	**7.95**	13.76	14.74	**15.71**
pps	2.46	14.72	17.16	**19.59**	33.90	36.32	**38.72**
fps	2.32	13.88	16.18	**18.47**	31.97	34.24	**36.51**

Table 4.6: Performance results of back-projection using the CBEA architecture for the two considered datasets using bilinear interpolation mode.

85.07%, and 92.56% can be reconstructed, respectively. The achieved frames per second using different numbers of SPEs in nearest neighbor and bilinear interpolation mode are given. The volume size in z-direction had to be adapted such that all slices are still in the FOV. It can be seen that proportional to the reduced number of necessary computations higher frame rates were achieved. Because sub-volumes at the border of the cylindrical FOV still include voxels lying outside of it, the overhead of our implementation increases, as theoretically expected, up to 5% for reconstructing 78.26% of the volume.

For the nearest neighbor interpolation mode the performance degrades slightly due to bandwidth limitation, when reconstructing only 85.07% or 78.26% (maximum speed-up factors were only 14.57 and 14.48, respectively). This results from the fact that for sub-volumes with increased voxel sizes the corresponding projection shadows will increase significantly. However, in bilinear interpolation mode this increased data transfer overhead was still hidden by the applied double buffering approach. Frame rates increased from 84.29 fps to 95.66 fps (nearest neighbor interpolation mode) and from 47.96 fps to 55.72 fps (bilinear interpolation mode).

In the next experiment we executed the filtering and the back-projection in parallel in a pipeline. The number of SPEs for filtering and back-projection has to be chosen statically before execution. Again, we examined the overall performance with

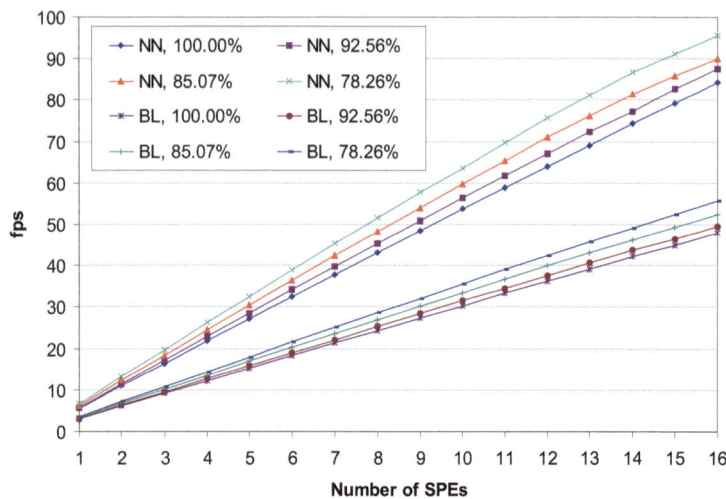

Figure 4.3: Field-of-view reconstruction with different voxel sizes. The achieved frames per second (fps) are given for reconstructions using Dataset (a). The percentage of the voxel volume that lies inside the FOV is given for each measurement. Frame rates are given for the two interpolation modes: nearest neighbor (NN) and bilinear (BL) interpolation.

both nearest neighbor and bilinear interpolation mode. Table 4.7 shows the corresponding results for various configurations. When only 8 SPEs of our dual Cell Blade are used, it is sufficient to execute the filtering with one SPE for maximum performance for both interpolation modes. The measured overall runtime reflects approximately the measured execution time of the back-projection with seven SPEs. Thus, filtering execution could be fully hidden behind the back-projection. In case of nearest neighbor interpolation more than 30 projections are processed per second, which still leverages an on-the-fly reconstruction using only one Cell processor. If one wants to achieve on-the-fly reconstruction also in bilinear interpolation mode at least two Cell processors have to be used (see Table 4.6). The achieved performance numbers of the overall pipelined execution validate that on-the-fly reconstruction is possible even in bilinear interpolation mode for all tested configurations of filtering and back-projection SPEs. However, maximum performance was only achieved when two SPEs are used for filtering the projection images in case of Dataset (b).

4.4 Summary

We have developed a parallelized and highly optimized implementation of the FDK method on the Cell processor. The achieved results demonstrate that a performance increase of an order of magnitude and more is achievable compared to recent high per-

| | Number of SPEs (filtering/back-projection) | | | | | |
| | using one Cell processor | | | using two Cell processors | | |
	1/7	2/6	3/5	1/15	2/14	3/13
Dataset (a), nearest neighbor interpolation						
Time [s]	**13.60**	15.75	18.83	7.39	**6.97**	7.45
pps	**30.44**	26.29	21.98	56.06	**59.43**	55.55
fps	**37.64**	32.52	27.18	69.33	**73.50**	68.70
Dataset (b), nearest neighbor interpolation						
Time [s]	**17.87**	20.66	24.69	14.78	**9.07**	9.67
pps	**30.39**	26.28	21.99	36.74	**59.90**	56.16
fps	**28.66**	24.78	20.74	34.64	**56.48**	52.95
Dataset (a), bilinear interpolation						
Time [s]	**24.04**	27.95	33.49	**11.44**	12.19	13.10
pps	**17.22**	14.81	12.36	**36.18**	33.95	31.61
fps	**21.30**	18.32	15.29	**44.74**	41.99	39.09
Dataset (b), bilinear interpolation						
Time [s]	**31.87**	36.99	44.28	16.21	**16.05**	17.22
pps	**17.04**	14.68	12.26	33.49	**33.84**	31.53
fps	**16.06**	13.84	11.56	31.58	**31.91**	29.73

Table 4.7: Overall pipelined execution of filtering and back-projection for the two considered datasets, bold numbers refer to optimum configurations.

formance general purpose computing platforms. We have shown that with our dual Cell Blade a complete FDK short-scan reconstruction (including weighting, filtering and back-projection) can be computed in 6.97 seconds (nearest neighbor interpolation) or 11.44 seconds (bilinear interpolation). It is a huge drawback of the Cell processor that it does not provide special hardware to efficiently compute the bilinear interpolation during projection access. We will see in Chapter 6 that other architectures outperform the Cell processor by providing special hardware circuits on-chip for this processing step.

Nevertheless, we have demonstrated that the Cell processor leverages cone-beam CT reconstructions on-the-fly for both interpolation modes, which means that all required computations are hidden behind the scan-time of the used scanner. Concerning real-time imaging, the achieved performance of the FDK method shows that there is still the possibility for computing additional pre-processing tasks such as beam hardening, truncation or scatter correction on the dual Cell Blade.

On the one hand the big advantage of the CBEA is its comprehensive programming control since it allows to implement well optimized code; on the other hand it is also one of its biggest drawbacks because it introduces high implementation complexity. We think that other hardware architectures such as graphics accelerators reveal their processing power with less implementation complexity, at least in the context of cone-beam image reconstruction.

Chapter 5

Standard Multi-Core Processors

For a long time, the performance of general-purpose processors could be improved by increasing clock frequency and instruction level parallelism (ILP). Nowadays, only diminished gains in performance can be reached by higher processor clock rates. This results from the difficulty to find enough parallelism in the instruction stream of a single process to keep higher performance processor cores busy. Another cause is the increasing gap between processor and main memory speed because the latency and the bandwidth of dynamic random access memory (DRAM) does not improve accordingly to processor operating frequencies. Finally, higher clock rates of general-purpose processors lead to dramatically increased problems in manufacturing, system design, and deployment. These three arguments, commonly referred to as the ILP wall, the memory wall and the power wall, respectively, have constituted much of the motivation for the advent of multi-core processors during the last few years.

5.1 Architecture

The amazing progress in VLSI design has led to the development of microprocessors consisting of several independent compute cores that can execute multiple application tasks in parallel. The cores belonging to one CPU often share certain levels of the on-chip memory hierarchy (e.g., on-chip L2 caches). These processors are commonly referred to as *multi-core* or even as *many-core CPUs*. Current CPU manufacturers such as Intel and AMD currently provide up to eight compute cores per CPU with forecasts predicting 32 and even more parallel cores per CPU chip.

In order to take advantage of the parallelism offered by multi-core systems software must run in several threads or processes. In most cases the application must be specifically written to utilize multiple threads. This also requires to identify an adequate algorithm structure which supports parallel execution.

Modern CPUs additionally feature so-called vector processing units (VPUs) to They provide the Streaming SIMD Extensions (SSE) which is the SIMD instruction set extension offered by CPUs from Intel and AMD. It allows to operate on four single precision floating-point numbers at once. Intel is doing research on processor chips such as the Larrabee processor, which will even extend the SIMD width and will therefore be able to process up to 16 single precision elements simultaneously [Seil 08].

Most modern compilers are able to automatically vectorize code in order to take advantage of the SIMD facilities of modern CPUs. The performance benefit of vectorization is better in parts of the program where many data elements are processed in the same way. Nowadays most compilers offer the possibility to directly assist the vectorization of the code by special built-in functions, which are commonly referred to as intrinsics. Intrinsics are convenient substitutes for one or more inline assembly instructions.

5.2   Feldkamp Algorithm

Using the supportive functionality of our RTK framework we implemented the processing chain of the FDK method as a pipeline architecture. Within this pipeline the filtering and the back-projection are executed in dedicated stages, respectively, using a different thread of control for each stage. This makes it possible to compute the corresponding filtering computations of projection $n + 1$ in parallel with the back-projection of projection n.

In order to do even more computations in parallel we further refined our implementation of both the filtering stage and the back-projection stage to make use of the Master/Worker parallelization pattern. When a projection image is processed by one of these stages, work packages are created, which are then processed by the corresponding worker threads of the stages. The number of worker threads was T_{FLT} for the filtering stage and T_{BP} for the back-projection stage.

5.2.1   Filtering

Using the frequency-based convolution approach as described in Section 2.2.2.1 each image row in a projection image can be processed independently from all other rows. It is thus easy to parallelize the computations for each projection image. We divided each projection image into T_{FLT} equally large chunks of consecutive rows and assigned each chunk to a different worker. This allowed us to compute the filtering of each chunk simultaneously on the available CPU cores.

In order to efficiently compute the necessary DFTs we used the complex 1-D FFT implementation of the Intel Integrated Performance Primitives (IPP) software library. Using the in-place functions `ippsFFTFwd_CToC_32f_I` and `ippsFFTInv_CToC_32f_I` for the forward and inverse transforms, respectively, we simultaneously convolve two image rows of a projection with the given filter kernel, where one image row defines the real input and the other one the imaginary input. During initialization of the FFTs we further used the `ippAlgHintFast` flag in order to select the fastest available implementation of the IPP library.

All additional computations have been implemented using intrinsics in order to compile a highly SIMD efficient code. The complex multiplication in Fourier domain was further optimized as our filter kernel was symmetric and, hence, its DFT contained only real values.

5.2.2 Back-Projection

In our parallel implementation of voxel-driven back-projection the volume is partitioned into T_{BP} disjoint sub-volumes and each sub-volume is assigned to one of the available worker threads (again cf. Figure 4.2). The voxels in a sub-volume are then projected onto the detector plane and updated with the corresponding interpolated projection values in the respective worker thread. Using this approach there is no need to synchronize voxel updates since each voxel is updated exactly once for each projection. All worker threads have read access to the complete projection image. This results in an efficient sharing of projection data between different worker threads through the cache hierarchy of the CPU.

In order to ensure that there are no competing write accesses to the volume we process the projection images sequentially in the order they are acquired. Therefore, any of the x, y, z loops of Algorithm 2 can be split into disjoint intervals to process them simultaneously.

We subdivided the whole volume in z-direction into T_{BP} sub-volumes consisting of several slice images of the volume. Each sub-volume is then assigned to one of the available worker threads. In theory this approach will scale linearly with the number of processor cores. Due to the large number of slice images N_z of the volume[1] this parallelization strategy will be sufficient to keep even the next-generation multi-core systems busy. Note that the overhead from thread creation is negligible because it happens only once during initialization of the worker threads.

Having found a suitable parallelization approach additional performance improvement can be achieved by vectorizing the code of each worker thread such that the SIMD facilities of the CPU are used in an efficient manner. Vectorization yields the highest performance gains in code parts where the same computations are performed on multiple data elements. As shown in Algorithm 2, the z- and y-loops do only compute the coordinate increments while the actual compute-intensive back-projection, including the corresponding bilinear interpolation for accessing the projection data, is done within the x-loop. This loop iterates over all voxels in one row of a slice (fixed y- and z-coordinate) and performs the same computations on each of them. We therefore concentrated on vectorizing this loop by processing four consecutive voxels in x-direction simultaneously using intrinsics.

While multi-threading was already supported by the RTK framework, all of the vectorization had to be done manually. Current VPUs have two inherent shortcomings. First, they cannot branch independently for individual elements of the vector and second, they cannot access memory in irregular patterns efficiently. During back-projection the necessary load instructions of the projection values expose both of these problems.

At the boundary of the FOV, one voxel may be projected outside of the detector while its neighbor's projection is still inside. If a voxel is projected outside of the detector its update is skipped and processing continues with the next one. In the vectorized version, these outliers had to be detected and stored in binary masks. The corresponding projection coordinates were set to $(0, 0)$ in order to avoid illegal memory accesses. Furthermore, the interpolated projection values for those voxels

---

[1] N_z is the number of voxels in z-direction

| | Vectorization | | |
	Compiler	Manual	Speedup
Dataset (a)	859.8	547.9	1.57
Dataset (b)	1135.5	722.9	1.57

Table 5.1: Single-threaded performance results of back-projection using the Xeon workstation with and without manual SIMD optimization (Intel compiler version 11.0.072).

were set to 0, resulting in a voxel increment with the value 0 which is equivalent to skipping the update.

Due to the projection geometry, neighboring voxels are usually not projected onto neighboring pixels in the projection image. This results in non-contiguous memory accesses when loading the projection values. Therefore, the projection values had to be read in a scalar manner and packed manually into SIMD vectors afterwards. Bilinear interpolation was then computed using these vectors on the VPU.

5.3 Results

In order to evaluate the performance of our implementation we used an off-the-shelf workstation from Fujitsu Siemens. It comprises two Intel Xeon Quad-Core processors (E5410) running at 2.33 GHz and having 16 GB of random access memory (RAM). The theoretical peak performance of this system is 74.6 Gflops.

We performed the measurements without doing the I/O transfers for loading the projection images from the hard disk or over the network. This is necessary in order to achieve runtime measurements that are not affected by I/O bandwidth limitations. We measured the performance of both the filtering and the back-projection step alone as well as their simultaneous overall execution. During our measurements we removed any outliers by taking only the best runtime out of three measurements.

The reconstruction has been done using a volume consisting of $512 \times 512 \times 512$ voxels. The voxel size was chosen accordingly to the geometry such that the whole volume is inside the FOV (see Appendix B for a description of the measurement setup). For our evaluations we compiled our implementation using the Intel compiler in version 11.0.072 and the IPP library in version 6.0.

We achieve a substantial performance improvement of the back-projection computations by manually optimizing the back-projection using SIMD intrinsics. This is shown in Table 5.1. Although the Intel compiler is known to be very good at auto-vectorization of program code, our manual SIMD optimization using compiler intrinsics results in a speedup of the back-projection execution time by 1.57. The observed speedup scales nearly linear with the number of cores used for back-projection.

Additionally the performance is substantially improved when using our paralleliza-tion approach for multi-core CPUs in combination with our manual SIMD optimized implementation variant. Table 5.2 shows the achieved performance for the filtering, the back-projection, and also for the overall execution of the pipeline. It can be seen that the back-projection performance scales nearly linear when using one, four or

Number of	Filtering		Back-Projection		Overall	
Threads	[s]	[pps]	[s]	[pps]	[s]	[pps]
Dataset (a), convolution length 2048						
1	5.8	72.0	547.9	0.8	553.8	0.8
4	3.5	118.8	138.0	3.0	140.0	3.0
8	7.9	52.7	70.6	5.9	72.1	5.8
Dataset (b), convolution length 4096						
1	14.5	37.5	722.9	0.8	736.9	0.7
4	5.6	97.9	182.0	3.0	186.0	2.9
8	6.7	81.0	93.6	5.8	96.5	5.6

Table 5.2: Performance results of filtering, back-projection and both combined (overall) on the Xeon workstation using one, four and eight cores.

eight cores of our dual quad-core Xeon workstation. The speedup with four and eight cores is 3.97 and 7.72, respectively. On the other hand, filtering performance is best using four cores for both datasets, although the achieved speedup does not scale with the number of cores used. The performance even degrades when using more than four cores due to synchronization overhead and due to the available main memory bandwidth.

Using all eight cores our implementation is able to process about 5.6 to 5.8 projections per second when executing filtering and back-projection (overall execution). Assuming that the execution time will scale linearly with the number of available cores and their clock frequency, one would thus need 32 cores running at 3.0 GHz to compute the reconstruction on-the-fly (30 pps). In a practical system, however, main memory bandwidth will most likely become a bottleneck.

5.4 Summary

We have developed a quite optimized implementation of the FDK method on general-purpose processors (Intel- or AMD-based). Both the filtering step and the back-projection step have been optimized for parallel execution on several processor cores. The FFTs have been implemented using the IPP software library. Our implementation of the back-projection includes manual vectorization of the code in order to make efficient use of the SIMD facilities of modern CPUs. We have shown that it is possible to achieve a speedup of 1.57 by a manual vectorization compared to the automatic vectorization of the compiler.

According to our results it is, however, nearly impossible to build systems that are able to accomplish on-the-fly reconstructions using only a few processor cores of current general-purpose processors.

Chapter 6

Graphics Accelerator Boards

While graphics accelerator boards are traditionally built for the gaming industry, nowadays these devices are usable for general computing tasks as well. GPUs are specialized for compute-intensive, highly parallel computations. In contrast to standard multi- or many-core architectures much more transistors are implemented for data processing rather than data caching and flow control. Hence, it is very appealing to use these architectures as acceleration platform for high-performance computing tasks in medical devices.

Two GPU vendors are currently offering GPU devices in the market supporting accelerated general purpose implementations: Nvidia and AMD/ATI. Since Nvidia has recently developed the fundamentally new easy-to-use computing paradigm *CUDA (Compute Unified Device Architecture)* for solving complex computational problems on the GPU, we focus on Nvidia devices in this thesis. The main contributions of this chapter have been presented at the IEEE Nuclear Science Symposium and Medical Imaging Conference 2007 [Sche 07b].

6.1 Architecture

CUDA offers a unified hardware and software solution for parallel computing on *CUDA*-enabled Nvidia GPUs supporting the standard C programming language together with high-performance computing numerical libraries[1]. This unveils the access to the processing power of graphics cards also for programmers that are not specialists in computer graphics. The implementation of the reconstruction task can now be done without knowing how to (ab)use the existing application programming interfaces for general-purpose computing; e.g., *OpenGL*[2], *DirectX*[3], or the *Brook* language[4].

Nvidia splits its GPUs into three different branches: GeForce, Quadro, and Tesla. GeForce devices target the gaming market. The professional graphics domain is addressed with Quadro devices, and Tesla provides the solution for high-performance computing. While each of these branches uses the same processor generation, the main difference refers to the type and amount of installed graphics memory (called

---

[1] http://www.nvidia.com/cuda
[2] http://www.khronos.org/opengl
[3] http://www.microsoft.com/windows/directx
[4] http://graphics.stanford.edu/projects/brookgpu

GPU	GeForce 8800 GTX	Tesla C870	GeForce GTX 280	Tesla C1060
Architecture	8 Series		200 Series	
Processor Cores	128		240	
Processor Clock [MHz]	1350		1296	
Gflops [MADD/MUL]	518		933	
Bus Width [bit]	384		512	
Memory Clock [MHz]	900	800	1107	800
Memory Bandwidth [GB/s]	86.4	76.8	141.7	102.4
Memory [GB]	0.768	1.500	1.000	4.000

Table 6.1: Technical overview of the considered graphics accelerator boards from Nvidia. The Tesla C870 is identical to the Quadro FX 5600. Likewise is the Tesla C1060 identical to the Quadro FX 5800. The difference between Quadro and Tesla is only in reliability of the memory and OpenGL support.

device memory in the following) together with the memory clock rate. For example, the memory chips of GeForce devices are usually over-clocked resulting in improved compute performance at the prize of less reliability. Occurring pixel errors on GeForce devices are considered to be of less importance due to their application in the gaming market. Quadro devices, on the other hand, target professional graphics applications and, thus, reliability of the memory is improved at the expense of lower memory clock rates. Finally, Tesla devices are mainly used in the high performance computing domain. The installed memory chips in Tesla devices provide the highest reliability. Tesla devices, however, support only computational applications, because all display adapters are removed from their boards, and OpenGL support is disabled.

Table 6.1 gives a technical overview of the high-end graphics accelerator boards, which are considered in this paper. In the following we distinguish two device series: the 8 series and the 200 series. We consider the GeForce 8800 GTX, the Quadro FX 5600, and the Tesla C870 GPUs from the 8 series and from the 200 series we consider the GeForce GTX 280, the Quadro FX 5800, and the Tesla C1060 GPUs. The theoretical peak performance increased by a factor of 1.8 between GPUs of the 8 series and GPUs of the 200 series. The memory bandwidth, however, only increased by a factor of 1.6 for the GeForce devices and by a factor of 1.3 for the Tesla and Quadro devices between the GPUs of the 8 series and the GPUs of the 200 series.

Modern GPUs in general have evolved into highly parallel, multi-threaded many-core processor architectures accompanied by graphics memory with very high bandwidth. The processor is build on a physically separated *device* and operates as a co-processor to the CPU (*host*). *CUDA* uses the SIMD programming model, since it provides an easy way to configure and run a huge amount of threads each operating on different data items. Each thread is executing the same program (*kernel*), which can be implemented as a C-function and is invoked by the host program via a special function call "syntax".

The considered GPUs offer 12 to 30 multi-processors each consisting of eight Stream Processors. A Stream Processor can compute three floating-point operations

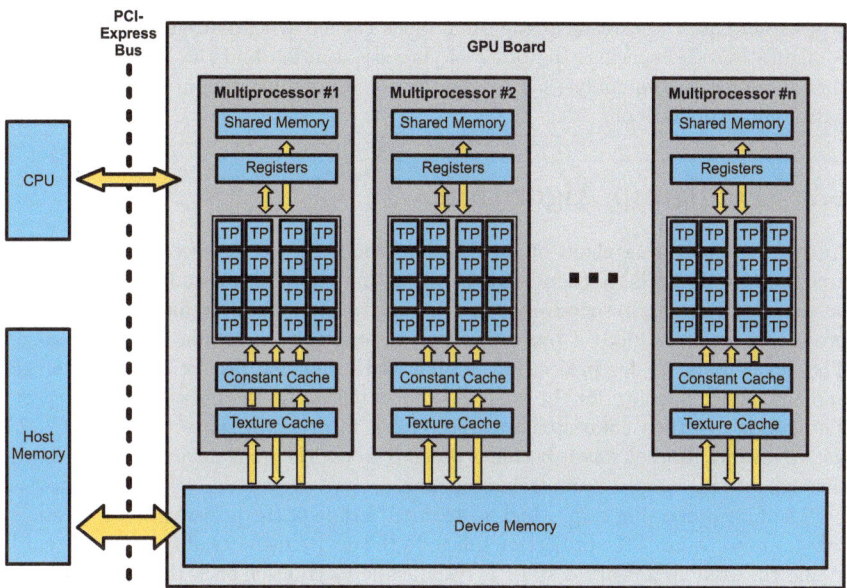

Figure 6.1: Architecture of modern Nvidia GPUs.

per clock cycle (one multiply-add and one multiplication), which results in a theoretical peak performance of 518 Gflops for the high-end GPUs of the 8 series, and 933 Gflops for the high-end GPUs of the 200 series.

Each multi-processor offers to its Stream Processors several resources, which have to be shared among them. Only a fixed number of registers is available limiting the maximum number of threads that can be executed simultaneously, and several data caches are available in order to reduce performance limitations due to memory bandwidth. Figure 6.1 gives an overview of the GPU architecture.

Stream Processors cannot access host memory directly, which requires to copy data to the device memory over the PCI-Express bus before kernel execution. A thread can read from and write to device memory directly (global memory access). For read-only memory accesses constant or texture caches can be used. The constant cache is limited by size and requires a special access pattern to achieve high performance. In contrast, texture memory is optimized for random access, and provides hardware-accelerated computation of bilinear and trilinear interpolation. Data items needed more than once by a thread (read/write) can be saved to register memory, which is used by the thread exclusively, or it can be transferred to shared memory. Like constant memory, shared memory requires a special access pattern in order to respect the GPU's memory architecture and therefore to deliver high bandwidth. Furthermore, it can only be shared and synchronized between a small number of threads, which have to be specified during kernel launch by a so called grid configuration. The threads of a kernel are grouped into 3-D arrays, which are called blocks, and blocks are grouped into a 2-D array, which is called grid. During the execution of a kernel only the threads of the same block can be synchronized. The grid-block configuration also specifies the order of thread execution and the identifier of each thread, which is commonly used to identify corresponding computation and/or the data item to operate on.

6.2   Feldkamp Algorithm

Again, the processing chain of the FDK method can be mapped to the pipeline architecture of the RTK framework by executing the filtering and back-projection on dedicated stages, respectively. In addition to the stages for filtering and back-projection we introduced a projection upload stage and a volume download stage. The device memory for projections is allocated inside the projection upload stage, and the device memory for the volume is allocated inside the back-projection stage. The stages are then connected single-threaded in order to share the same *CUDA device context*. In that way it becomes possible to use the same device data structures throughout the complete processing pipeline.

The first processing step, which is executed inside of the projection upload stage, takes care to transfer the projection image to the device memory of the graphics card. While the volume download stage is responsible to transfer back the volume to the host memory, the filtering and the back-projection are executed between the upload and download stages, respectively.

6.2.1   Filtering

The filtering stage is implemented using the *CUFFT library* of the *CUDA package* to compute the convolution with the given filter kernel. This library supports the calculation of complex FFT. All necessary computations are mapped to several successive *CUDA kernel* executions: data rearrangement to complex format, zero-padding, batched FFT, multiplication with the DFT of the filter kernel, batched IFFT, and data rearrangement to the original format. Each *CUDA kernel* computes all rows of a complete projection image simultaneously in order to make efficient use of the multiprocessors on the graphics card.

6.2.2   Back-Projection

In order to compute the voxel-driven back-projection on the GPU we store the complete volume in global device memory, because in *CUDA*, global memory is the only memory type that can be accessed for writing. The back-projection for a projection image is computed as soon as the filtering stage has finished the corresponding convolution task.

Our back-projection implementation uses a loop on the host (CPU) to prepare and to control the execution of the GPU program code, which is commonly referred to as the kernel program, on the device (GPU). Algorithm 5 gives an overview of our implementation strategy: projection images are streamed to the GPU and are processed immediately while the volume keeps fixed in device memory. We further store each projection matrix $\check{P}_i$ in constant device memory and bind a texture context

---

Algorithm 5: Pseudo-code of our GPU-based back-projection implementation.

Input: N_p projection images $\mathbf{I}_i$, $0 \leq i < N_p$
Input: N_p projection matrices $\check{\mathbf{P}}_i$, $0 \leq i < N_p$
Data: volume $\mathbf{V}$ consisting of $N_x \times N_y \times N_z$ voxels stored in device memory

1 **Host:**

2 **for** $(i = 0; i < N_p; i = i + 1)$ **do**
3   Load memory of $\mathbf{I}_i$ to device memory;
4   Load $\check{\mathbf{P}}_i$ to constant device memory;
5   Call Kernel;
6 **end**
7 Download volume $\mathbf{V}$ to host memory;

8 **Kernel:**

9 Compute $\check{x}$ and $\check{z}$ coordinate of voxel;   // cf. Figure 6.2
  // Compute base-increment
10 $r_{xz} = \check{\mathbf{P}}_i[0,0] \cdot \check{x} + \check{\mathbf{P}}_i[0,2] \cdot \check{z} + \check{\mathbf{P}}_i[0,3]$;
11 $s_{xz} = \check{\mathbf{P}}_i[1,0] \cdot \check{x} + \check{\mathbf{P}}_i[1,2] \cdot \check{z} + \check{\mathbf{P}}_i[1,3]$;
12 $t_{xz} = \check{\mathbf{P}}_i[2,0] \cdot \check{x} + \check{\mathbf{P}}_i[2,2] \cdot \check{z} + \check{\mathbf{P}}_i[2,3]$;
13 **for** $(\check{y} = 0; \check{y} < N_y; \check{y} = \check{y} + 1)$ **do**
14    $r = r_{xz} + \check{\mathbf{P}}_i[0,1] \cdot \check{y}$;
15    $s = s_{xz} + \check{\mathbf{P}}_i[1,1] \cdot \check{y}$;
16    $t = t_{xz} + \check{\mathbf{P}}_i[2,1] \cdot \check{y}$;

17    $\check{u} = \frac{r}{t}$;   // Dehomogenize
18    $\check{v} = \frac{s}{t}$;   // Dehomogenize
19    $\mu = \frac{1}{t^2}$;   // Distance weight

20    $\mathbf{V}[\check{x}, \check{y}, \check{z}] = \mathbf{V}[\check{x}, \check{y}, \check{z}] + \mu \, \text{texfetch}(\mathbf{I}_i, \check{u}, \check{v})$;   // Accumulate
21 **end**

---

to the projection data. Texture memory is not only optimized for fast random memory accesses, it further enables a performance improvement by using the texture hardware of the GPU either for nearest neighbor interpolation or hardware-accelerated bilinear interpolation.

Then we invoke our back-projection kernel on the graphics device. Each thread of the kernel computes the back-projection for all voxels of a certain column in a volume slice (see Figure 6.2). Instead of calculating for each voxel the whole matrix-vector product (nine multiply-add operations), six multiply-add operations can be avoided in the innermost loop by incrementing the homogeneous coordinates with the appropriate column of $\check{\mathbf{P}}_i$ for neighboring voxels in y-direction.

The incremental back-projection implementation does not only reduce the number of arithmetic operations (cf. Section 2.2.3) but it also reduces the register usage of the corresponding kernel program to only ten registers (see Figure 6.3).

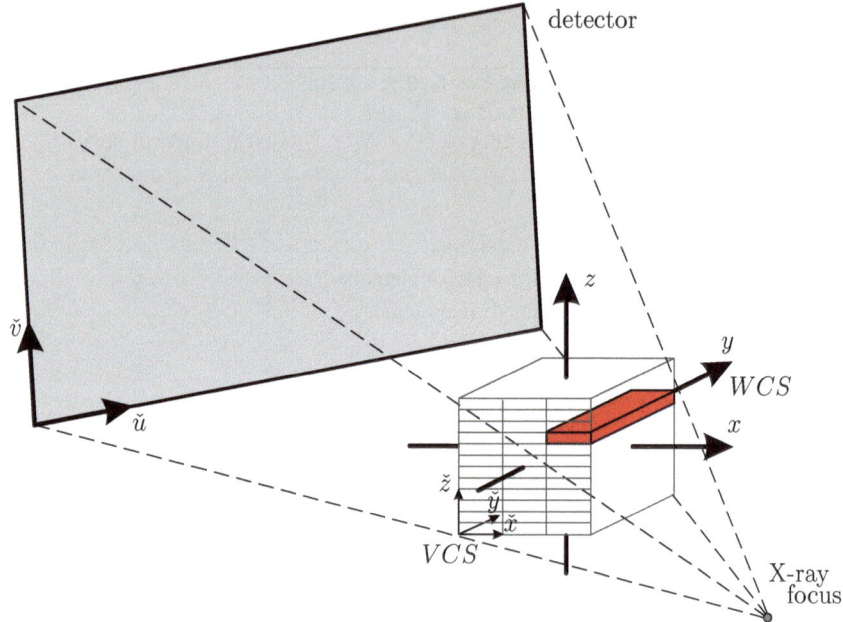

Figure 6.2: Perspective geometry of the C-arm device (the $\check{v}$-axis and $\check{z}$-axis are not necessarily parallel) together with the parallelization strategy of our back-projection implementation on the GPU using $CUDA$ (the $\check{x}$-$\check{z}$ plane is divided into several blocks to specify a grid configuration, and each thread of a corresponding block processes all voxels in $\check{y}$-direction).

Using more than ten registers would reduce the number of threads that can be executed simultaneously by the kernel program. The multiprocessor warp occupancy can be used as an indicator of the ability to hide latencies of device memory accesses behind arithmetic computations (see Figure 6.3). A higher warp occupancy will, therefore, more likely result in a better thread scheduling on the device. While the threads of a warp have to wait for the completion of a memory transfer the threads of another warp can use the waiting time for computations. More registers are available per multi-processor on GPUs of the 200 series. This significantly relaxes the requirement on register usage.

The increased number of registers on GPUs of the 200 series makes it possible to loop over a few projection images in the inner-most loop (see Algorithm 6). Using this approach, a huge amount of previously required global memory accesses can be avoided. For example, looping over two projections in the inner-loop requires only half as much global memory accesses and looping over three projections even requires only one-third of the required global memory accesses.

In order to achieve high memory bandwidth on GPUs of the 200 series the volume memory layout had to be padded appropriately. The memory architecture of these devices is taken into account by padding each row such that its total size in bytes is

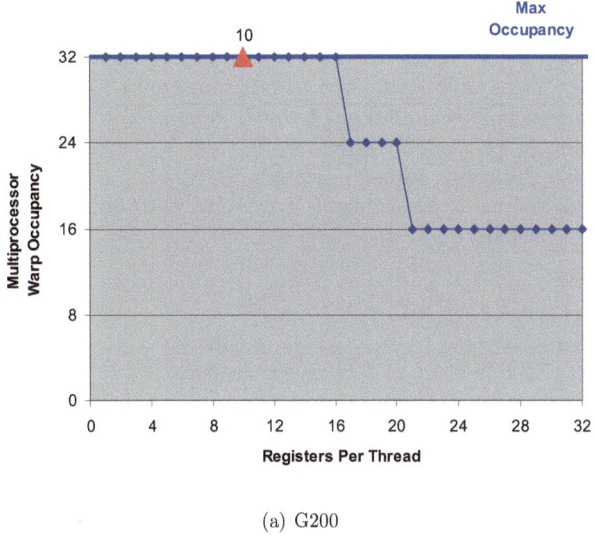

(a) G200

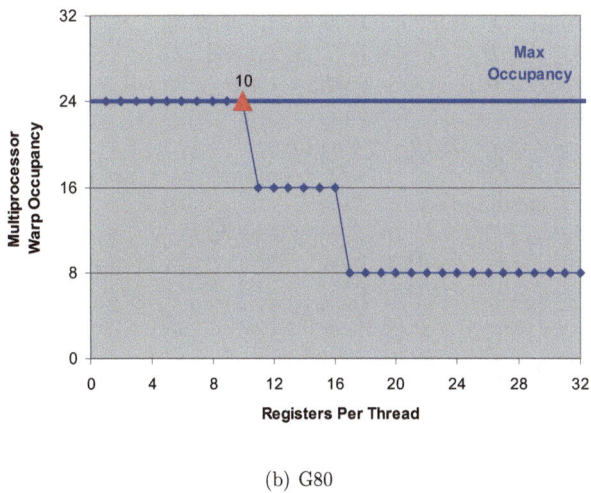

(b) G80

Figure 6.3: Dependency of the multiprocessor warp occupancy on the register usage for the considered GPUs of the 200 series (a), and the considered GPUs of the 8 series (b). Our *CUDA* implementation uses only 10 registers. Register usage has been much more important on the G80 device series due to the lower number of available registers per multi-processor.

Algorithm 6: Pseudo-code of the GPU-based back-projection that
loops additionally over several projections.

Input: N_p projection images $\mathbf{I}_i$, $0 \leq i < N_p$
Input: N_p projection matrices $\check{\mathbf{P}}_i$, $0 \leq i < N_p$
Input: Projection sequence size N_{seq}
Data: volume $\mathbf{V}$ consisting of $N_x \times N_y \times N_z$ voxels stored in device
memory

1 **Host:**

2 **for** $(i = 0; i < N_p; i = i + N_{seq})$ **do**
3   **for** $(j = i; j < i + N_{seq}; j = j + 1)$ **do**
4   Load memory of $\mathbf{I}_i$ to device memory;
5   Load $\check{\mathbf{P}}_i$ to constant device memory;
6   **end**
7   Call Kernel;
8 **end**

9 **Kernel:**

10 Compute voxel $\check{x}$ and $\check{z}$ coordinate;
   // Compute base-increments for each projection
11 **for** $(j = i; j < i + N_{seq}; j = j + 1)$ **do**
12    $r_{xz}[j] = \check{\mathbf{P}}_j[0,0] \cdot \check{x} + \check{\mathbf{P}}_j[0,2] \cdot \check{z} + \check{\mathbf{P}}_j[0,3]$;
13    $s_{xz}[j] = \check{\mathbf{P}}_j[1,0] \cdot \check{x} + \check{\mathbf{P}}_j[1,2] \cdot \check{z} + \check{\mathbf{P}}_j[1,3]$;
14    $t_{xz}[j] = \check{\mathbf{P}}_j[2,0] \cdot \check{x} + \check{\mathbf{P}}_j[2,2] \cdot \check{z} + \check{\mathbf{P}}_j[2,3]$;
15 **end**
16 **for** $(\check{y} = 0; \check{y} < N_y; \check{y} = \check{y} + 1)$ **do**
17    $v_{tmp} = 0.0$;   // Temporary back-projection result
     // Unrolled:
18   **for** $(j = i; j < i + N_{seq}; j = j + 1)$ **do**
19       $r = r_{xz}[j] + \check{\mathbf{P}}_j[0,1] \cdot \check{y}$;
20       $s = s_{xz}[j] + \check{\mathbf{P}}_j[1,1] \cdot \check{y}$;
21       $t = t_{xz}[j] + \check{\mathbf{P}}_j[2,1] \cdot \check{y}$;
22       $\check{u} = \frac{r}{t}$;   // Dehomogenize
23       $\check{v} = \frac{s}{t}$;   // Dehomogenize
24       $\mu = \frac{1}{t^2}$;   // Distance weight
25       $v_{tmp} = v_{tmp} + \mu \, \text{texfetch}(\mathbf{I}_j, \check{u}, \check{v})$;   // Accumulate
26   **end**
27    $\mathbf{V}[\check{x}, \check{y}, \check{z}] = \mathbf{V}[\check{x}, \check{y}, \check{z}] + v_{tmp}$;   // Final accumulation
28 **end**

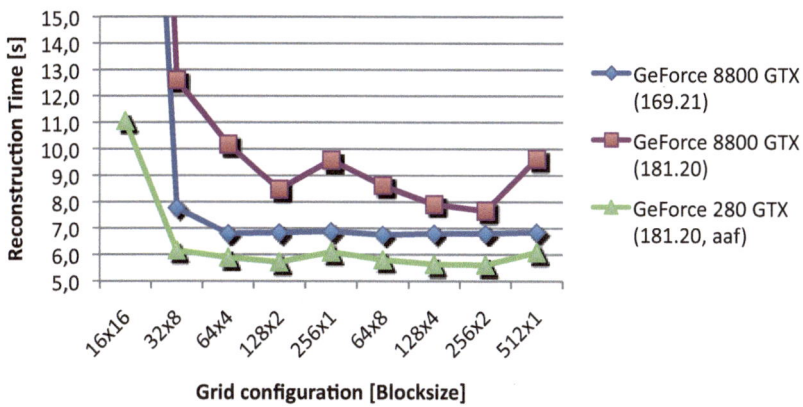

Figure 6.4: Execution time for different grid configurations.

a multiple of 32, but not by 512. In the following we call the adaption of the memory layout address aliasing fix (aaf). This is necessary in order to avoid problems due to partition camping, which can degrade device memory bandwidth drastically on GPUs of the 200 series. Unfortunately, the provided *CUDA* memory allocation routines do not care about this issue automatically (including CUDA version 2.1). While this behavior is not documented by Nvidia the mentioned optimization is not obvious to the programmer.

6.3   Results

In order to evaluate the filtering and back-projection performance of our GPU implementation, we installed three different workstations each equipped with two graphics accelerators. In each workstation we used an *Intel Xeon* Quad-core processor (E5440) running at 2.83 GHz. We show results obtained with six different graphics accelerators from Nvidia, namely the *GeForce 8800 GTX*, the *GeForce GTX 280*, the *Quadro FX 5600*, the *Tesla C870*, the *Quadro FX 5800*, and the *Tesla C1060*.

The performance has been evaluated with the same datasets and with the same configurations which have already been used in Sections 5.3 and 4.3 (see Appendix B for a detailed description).

It is very important to choose an appropriate grid configuration. The grid configuration influences both the global memory access pattern and the texture cache usage. Our experiments show that it is more important to optimize the global memory accesses than optimizing the texture cache usage (see Figure 6.4). It can be seen that it is important to have at least 64 to 128 threads in a block in x-direction, otherwise reconstruction performance is significantly degraded. This is more important on GPUs of the 8 series as can be seen in Figure 6.4 as well. For both device series, a grid configuration of 256×2 has been demonstrated to be optimal. It is an interesting

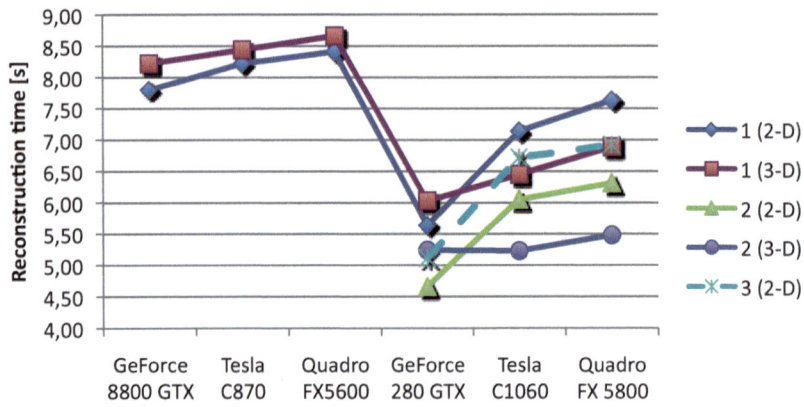

Figure 6.5: Comparison of back-projection performance when using a loop over several projections in the inner-most back-projection loop.

observation that less reconstruction performance is achieved on GPUs of the 8 series using device driver 181.20 compared to the performance that is achievable using device driver 169.21. In addition to that the grid configuration significantly influences the reconstruction performance on devices of the 8 series using the more recent driver.

In the next step we fix the grid configuration and evaluate how the back-projection performance is influenced when looping over a few projection images in the inner-most loop (see Algorithm 6). Figure 6.5 shows the achieved performance results. Unfortunately, GPUs of the 8 series could not execute any back-projection kernel where the inner-most loop has been unrolled due to their limited number of GPU registers.

In this regard, a rectification-based approach has the potential to further improve the reconstruction speed [Ridd 06] since it would require fewer computations and projection matrix accesses. This would allow to implement unrolled loops over projections in the inner-most back-projection loop also for GPUs of the 8 series, and even more unrolled loops for GPUs of the 200 series without an increase in register usage. We, however, intentionally avoided rectification-based approaches, as was already outlined in Section 2.2.2.2.

It can further be seen in Figure 6.5 that the graphics driver follows different driver paths for each branch of devices. For example, it is more efficient to save all projections in one flattened 2-D texture than in a 3-D texture using the GeForce devices. Using Quadro or Tesla devices, however, it is more efficient to use a 3-D texture. Unrolling the inner-most loop over two projection images proved to be a very efficient optimization trick. The bandwidth limitation of back-projection is reduced due to the saved global memory accesses.

In the following we used for each device its optimal implementation which can easily be extracted from Figure 6.5. For example, we unroll the inner-most loop twice for GPUs of the 200 series, and do no unrolling on GPUs of the older 8 series because

Hardware	Filtering		Back-Projection		Overall	
	[s]	pps	[s]	pps	[s]	pps
Dataset (a), convolution length 2048						
Quadro FX 5600	2,6	158,6	8,3	50,2	12,0	34,4
Tesla C870	2,3	181,6	8,1	51,4	11,4	36,3
GeForce 8800 GTX	2,2	184,8	7,5	55,0	10,7	38,6
Quadro FX 5800	1,6	265,4	5,4	76,4	7,9	52,3
Tesla C1060	1,3	309,0	5,2	79,3	7,3	57,1
GeForce GTX 280	1,5	281,6	4,6	89,2	7,1	58,5
Dataset (b), convolution length 4096						
Quadro FX 5600	6,6	82,9	11,5	47,3	19,8	27,5
Tesla C870	6,0	91,0	11,2	48,5	18,5	29,4
GeForce 8800 GTX	5,9	91,9	10,6	51,3	17,8	30,5
Quadro FX 5800	3,9	138,5	8,5	63,9	13,5	40,2
Tesla C1060	3,5	156,5	8,2	66,1	12,6	43,1
GeForce GTX 280	3,6	153,0	6,7	80,7	11,4	47,5

Table 6.2: GPU performance results of filtering and back-projection for the considered devices of the 8 series and 200 series.

it has not been possible on the these devices. In Table 6.2, we show the timing measurements for the filtering, back-projection, and also for the overall execution for each device under consideration. We also give the numbers of projections that can be processed per second (pps).

Comparing the measured results of the *Tesla* and *Quadro* devices we achieved slightly better reconstruction speed for the *Tesla* devices, although *Tesla* and *Quadro* devices of the same GPU series are based upon the same hardware components. We think that this difference results from overheads caused by frequent thread context changes on the *Quadro* devices since we also used the *Quadro* device as the primary display adapter in our test systems.

The Fourier-based filtering is not affected by memory bandwidth, and between GPUs of the 8 series and the 200 series the theoretical speedup of 1.8 due to computing resources is nearly reached. This is, however, not the case for the back-projection. The difference in execution times for the *Quadro* and *GeForce* follows roughly the difference in device memory bandwidth when no loop unrolling is applied. This is an indicator that our back-projection performance is bandwidth-limited. In this regard, the loop over multiple projections in the innermost back-projection loop proved to be a very effective optimization. Thus, the increase in performance between the two considered GPU series does not follow the speed-up in device memory bandwidth any more. Instead the reached speed-up factor is right in the middle between the speed-up that is possible due to the increased amount of computing resources and due to the higher memory bandwidth.

Under the assumption that practical cone-beam CT scanners acquire 30 projections per second, all considered devices allow to compute the FDK reconstruction on-the-fly. However, in an on-the-fly reconstruction for Dataset (b) a small number of projection buffers would be required for the Quadro and Tesla devices of the 8 series since their reconstruction performance is a little bit under the required 30 projections per second. On the other hand, the GPUs of the 200 series allow to implement even more required preprocessing steps on the GPU while still running an on-the-fly reconstruction.

6.4   Summary

We have presented an optimized CUDA-based implementation of the FDK method. The achieved performance leverages cone-beam CT reconstructions on-the-fly, which means that we can hide all required computations behind the scan-time of the used X-ray acquisition device.

We have shown that a straight-forward implementation of back-projection is limited by device memory bandwidth. We have additionally developed an implementation that overcomes this limitation by looping over multiple projections in the innermost back-projection loop. The workaround is, however, expensive in regard to register usage such that it could only be applied to the GPU devices of the 200 series and above.

In contrast to traditional implementation approaches using OpenGL and shading languages, for example, the CUDA architecture enables the non-graphics programmer to implement efficient GPU code for general-purpose computations in a more simplified and appropriate way. With respect to the implementation of the FDK method the CUDA-based approach has required much less implementation effort than an optimized CBEA-based implementation.

Chapter 7

FPGA-Based Hardware

Besides off-the-shelf graphics cards, reconfigurable hardware has been gaining attention in the field of massively parallel high-performance computing as well. Several computer manufacturers offer FPGA-based accelerator components together with dedicated libraries in order to speed up the execution of numerically intensive codes. Such hardware components are particularly appropriate for applications in the signal processing domain such as image or video compression, for instance.

Generally speaking, an FPGA is a dynamically reconfigurable microchip that covers logical hardware blocks (e.g., look-up tables), arithmetic units (e.g., multiply-add blocks), as well as I/O functionality [Meye 08]. Todays FPGA designs typically run at clock rates of 100 MHz up to 500 MHz. An FPGA must be loaded with an appropriate *firmware* (also known as *bitstream*) before it provides its functionality. The generation of such a bitstream is commonly a complex process that involves a series of software tools covering the steps of netlist synthesis and place-and-route, amongst others. However, the details of the firmware generation process are far beyond the scope of this thesis. In short, a higher-level representation of the hardware functionality (typically given as VHDL code or as Verilog code) is turned into the actual firmware to be loaded into the FPGA.

The main contributions of this chapter have been presented in part at the Symposium on Simulation Techniques 2005 [Sche 05].

7.1   Architecture of the *ImageProX* Hardware

As an example of an FPGA-based accelerator hardware, we focus on the *ImageProX* (*image processing accelerator*) board that has been developed at Siemens Healthcare and was released in 2006. The *ImageProX* board uses either a 64 bit PCI interface (66 MHz) or a 64 bit PCI-X interface (133 MHz) to connect to the host PC. It covers nine Xilinx Virtex-4 FPGAs (1× Virtex-4 SX55, 8× Virtex-4 SX35), each of which is equipped with up to 1 GB of external DDR2 SDRAM memory. The *ImageProX* board comprises two identically organized rings of four Virtex-4 SX35 chips each, with the even more powerful Virtex-4 SX55 FPGA representing the core control and interface unit of the design.

Figure 7.1 clearly shows the *ImageProX* architecture with its nine Xilinx FPGAs. See [Heig 07] for further architecture details.

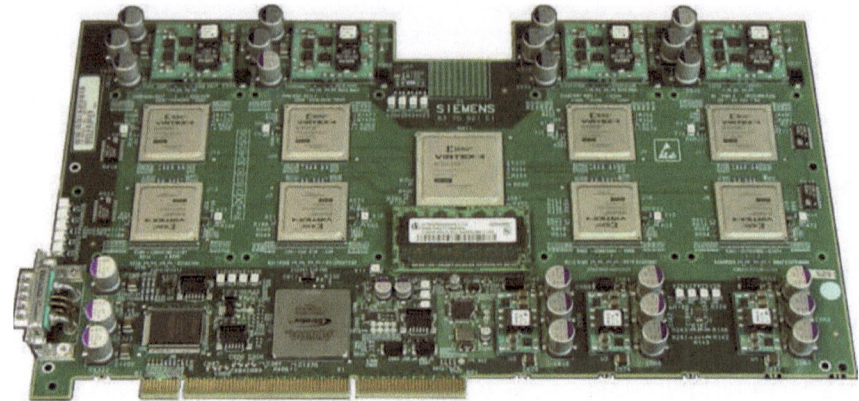

Figure 7.1: FPGA-based *ImageProX* accelerator board.

Assuming a system clock rate of 200 MHz and counting the aforementioned arithmetic units of the FPGAs only (while ignoring that standard FPGA logic can also be used for computing purposes), *ImageProX* offers a peak performance of more than 800 Giga operations per second. It must be pointed out that FPGAs currently offer fixed-point arithmetic only. If, however, floating-point arithmetic is required for the sake of numerical accuracy, floating-point units must be built "manually" using the available fixed-point units. This typically leads to inefficient designs that cannot cope with compute architectures that natively support floating-point operations.

7.2   Feldkamp Algorithm

Our *ImageProX*-based implementation of the FDK method covers the two essential steps of filtering the rows of each individual projection as well as back-projecting the filtered projection data into the volume.

7.2.1   Filtering

As was already mentioned above, a significant downside to our FPGA-based approach is that it is no longer possible to use floating-point arithmetic, as is the case for conventional CPU-based implementations, for example. Consequently, it is necessary to realize the whole processing chain of the convolution using fixed-point numbers instead. In order to simulate the effects of fixed-point calculations on the accuracy of the final numerical results, we have developed a highly flexible and bit-accurate software prototype of the hardware design. It covers both the FFT routines as well as different scaling strategies of the involved fixed-point data types. Additionally, various hardware restrictions of the FPGA architecture had to be considered throughout the simulation task to achieve optimal performance and to meet the resource restrictions on the chips.

In order to simulate the convolution chain using fixed-point data types, we based our software prototype on the *SystemC* library[1]. This library offers the possibility to use variables with limited accuracy, thus facilitating the simulation of configurable bit-widths of the involved data types. The simulation itself can be divided into two different parts. First, the involved fixed-point FFT and IFFT computations have to be simulated bit-accurately with different input and output bit-widths and with an appropriate internal scaling strategy. In a second step, the intermediate computing stages have to be implemented taking into account the input and output bit-widths of the FFT and the IFFT. In order to keep the input signals properly scaled within the FFT computations, we selected two different approaches. We will refer to them as *block floating-point mode* and *unscaled precision mode*, respectively. In the following, we are looking for a fixed-point implementation on the *ImageProX* board that employs the FFT cores of the Xilinx CoreGen Library[2].

7.2.1.1 Block Floating-Point Mode

In the block floating-point mode, the complexity of scaling is integrated almost completely into the FFTs. As the data moves from stage to stage through the calculation, the magnitudes of the numbers in the sequence generally increase, which means that they can be properly scaled by right shifts. In this case, we test after each butterfly computation, whether an overflow has occurred. Whenever an overflow has occurred, the entire sequence (part of which will be new results, part of which will be entries yet to be processed) is shifted right by one bit and the computations are continued at the point at which the overflow has occurred. The block exponent records the number of applied shifts. It can be shown that there are only two overflow events possible within each FFT stage [Welc 69]. One advantage of this approach is that only a minimum of computations is required for scaling purposes in between the FFT computations.

The processing chain looks as follows. The 16 bit entries of the block-scaled input vectors[3] are padded with zeros to a length of 24 bit. Then, the FFT and the multiplication with the DFT of the filter kernel (32 bit block-scaled fixed-point numbers in our case) are performed. After the multiplication, the resulting numbers are 56 bit wide. We simply chop off the trailing 32 bits to apply the IFFT with again 24 bits on input. Finally, the results of the IFFT (24 bit each) are truncated to 16 bits for the output. For improved accuracy, we also tried out this approach with 35 as the input and output bit-width of both the FFT and the IFFT.

7.2.1.2 Unscaled Precision Mode

The scaling inside the FFT blocks is done differently in unscaled precision mode. Within each FFT stage, the bit-width of the results is increased by one. Therefore, during the computations, overflows cannot occur anymore. Analogously, this strategy

---

[1] See http://www.systemc.org.

[2] See http://www.xilinx.com.

[3] The complex value integer pairs of the input vector of an FFT block are represented with a single scale factor (block exponent) that is shared among all complex value integer pairs of that vector.

can be understood as introducing a global right shift before each stage without loosing the least significant bit. In contrast to the previous approach, this technique exhibits the disadvantage that the output sequence of the FFT may not be properly scaled anymore. Therefore, a more advanced scaling technique is needed in between the FFT and the IFFT block. We will refer to our implemented technique as *dynamic scaling*. During the dynamic scaling, the minimum number of irrelevant bits to the right of the sign bit of all numbers of the current data vector is computed. Afterwards, all vector elements are left-shifted by that number, and the block exponent is adapted appropriately. This results in a simplification of the hardware implementation of the FFT and IFFT routines, which in turn leverages their optimization for processing speed. The loss of efficiency in the dynamic scaling stages in between the FFT and the IFFT can easily be accounted for by the use of pipelining in the hardware implementation [Henn 03].

The processing chain now involves the computation of the FFT of input vectors of (zero-padded) 24 bit numbers using the unscaled precision mode. Therefore, the output bit-width after the FFT block[4] is 37 bit for the case of a 4K convolution (or 38 bit for the case of an 8K convolution). Due to FPGA hardware constraints of the used Xilinx chips related to the internal architecture of multipliers, the values of the output sequence are truncated to 35 bits, and a dynamic rescaling is performed right before the multiplication stage. The 67 bit wide entries of the resulting product vector (recall that the DFT of the filter sequence is given as a vector of 32 bit numbers) are truncated to 36 bits, and a dynamic rescaling is performed again. Then, the vector entries are truncated to the input bit-width of the IFFT (i.e., 24 bit). After the IFFT, a final dynamic rescaling is introduced before truncating the vector entries to the required output bit-width with minimal loss of accuracy.

7.2.1.3 Implementation

The final FPGA implementation was realized at Siemens Healthcare. The filtering stage is completely implemented as part of the Virtex-4 SX55 firmware and runs fully pipelined at a clock rate of 200 MHz. Since two projection rows are filtered simultaneously, this yields a processing speed of 400 Mega samples per second. With each sample being represented as a 16 bit fixed-point value, the filtering stage is thus able to process 800 MByte of projection data per second, which exceeds the peak bandwidth of the 66 MHz PCI interface and is close to the peak bandwidth of about 1 GByte per second of the 133 MHz PCI-X interface. Consequently, the filtering stage does not represent a data processing bottleneck. The FFT/IFFT blocks of the *ImageProX* filtering stage are generated using the Xilinx CoreGen library. Internally, a block floating-point format is employed in oder to meet the size restrictions of the FPGA chip.

---

[4] Using the unscaled precision mode of the Xilinx CoreGen library the output data width of the FFT blocks equals (input data width + $\log_2$(point size) + 1).

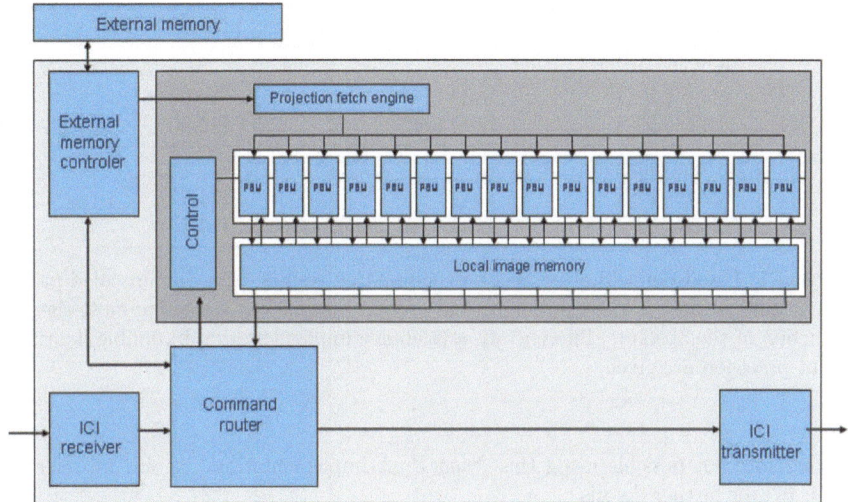

Figure 7.2: Design of the back-projection stage within an SX35 FPGA.

7.2.2 Back-Projection

A sophisticated FPGA-based high-performance implementation of the FDK method is out of scope of this thesis. Nevertheless, we briefly outline the final implementation that has been done at Siemens Healthcare.

The back-projection is accomplished simultaneously by the eight Virtex-4 SX35 FPGAs. As is the case for both the Cell-based as well as the GPU-based implementations, the volume is being reconstructed in a blockwise manner. In a typical reconstruction setting with nearly optimal load balancing, each of the SX35 chips will store approximately the same number of projection images in its external SDRAM memory. Hence, each of the SX35 chips is responsible for back-projecting its own set of projection images into the current volume block.

Analogous to the filtering engine, the back-projection design is fully pipelined as well, such that a peak speed of about 25 Giga back-projection steps per second can be achieved in theory: 200 MHz × 8 SX35 FPGAs × 16 back-projection pipelines per SX35 FPGA. Figure 7.2 illustrates the design of the back-projection stage within an SX35 chip; 16 so-called *parallel back-projection units (PBUs)* simultaneously read a portion of the FPGA-internal memory that stores the portion of the current projection to be back-projected into the volume. The current volume block to be written is kept in a separate portion of FPGA-internal memory (denoted as *Local image memory* in Figure 7.2).

It is important to point out that the back-projection phase can only start as soon as all projections (or at least a significantly large portion of projections) has been transferred into the FPGA-external memories. An on-the-fly reconstruction that immediately processes and back-projects a projection as soon as it becomes available

Unscaled precision	Head phantom [bits]	Thorax phantom [bits]
4K convolution		
23 bit FFT	14 (14.98)	15 (15.00)
24 bit FFT	14 (14.98)	15 (15.00)
8K convolution		
22 bit FFT	14 (14.84)	14 (14.95)
24 bit FFT	14 (14.84)	14 (14.95)

Table 7.1: Fixed-point filtering accuracy simulation results using the unscaled precision scaling strategy. The minimum (and average) number of vanishing most significant bits of the absolute difference to a reference implementation in double floating-point precision are given.

is therefore not possible using this *ImageProX* implementation. Again, we refer to [Heig 07] for further details.

7.3 Results

7.3.1 Simulation of Bit-Accurate Filtering

Throughout the evaluation of the accuracy of our different scaling approaches, we used projection images that are generated with the simulation tool *DRASIM* that had been provided by Siemens Healthcare. We used two analytic phantom descriptions: the Head Phantom and the Thorax Phantom. Descriptions of these phantoms can be found on the FORBILD website[5]. In order to measure the accuracy of our results, we compared each computed signal to the corresponding one that was computed using a reference code based on double-precision floating-point arithmetic using a standard Shepp-Logan filter kernel. For the bit comparison of two numbers, we counted the number of vanishing most significant bits of their absolute difference. Then, for each result vector, both the minimum and the average of the determined corresponding leading bits are used.

Table 7.1 shows the measured accuracies using the unscaled precision arithmetic. The results demonstrate that this approach yields very good accuracy in comparison with the double-precision floating-point results. The measured accuracy does not change even when we tweak the input bit width of the FFTs to match optimally the hardware restrictions both in the 4K convolution case with an input bit-width of 23 bits and in the 8K convolution case with an input bit-width of 22 bits.

Because of its advantageous structure with regard to hardware implementation and resources on the ImageProX board, we turned our attention more on the block floating-point arithmetic. In Table 7.2, the measured accuracies using the block floating-point scaling strategy are given. The achieved accuracy is about 9 to 10 bits both for 24 bit and 35 bit FFT structures. The loss of several valid bits results

---

[5] http://www.imp.uni-erlangen.de/phantoms

Block floating-point	Head phantom [bits]	Thorax phantom [bits]
4K convolution		
24 bit FFT	10 (10.98)	11 (11.00)
35 bit FFT	10 (11.38)	11 (11.35)
4K convolution (improved)		
24 bit FFT	11 (11.98)	
35 bit FFT	14 (14.98)	
8K convolution		
24 bit FFT	10 (10.44)	9 (9.96)
35 bit FFT	10 (10.65)	10 (10.43)

Table 7.2: Fixed-point filtering accuracy simulation results using the block floating-point scaling strategy. The minimum (and average) number of vanishing most significant bits of the absolute difference to a reference implementation in double floating-point precision are given.

	Back-Projection		Overall	
	[s]	pps	[s]	pps
Dataset (a)	3.9	107.3	11.2	36.9
Dataset (b)	4.4	124.5	15.0	36.3

Table 7.3: Reconstruction performance results of back-projection and overall reconstruction including filtering for the *ImageProX* board.

from the bit truncation after the multiplication with the DFT of the filter sequence. Therefore, we extended the scaling strategy of the block floating-point mode after the multiply stage by performing first a truncation to 35 bits and second by a dynamic rescaling afterwards. Then, the sequence is truncated to match the input size of the IFFT. Now, the results are as expected for the 35 bit case, but not much better for the 24 bit case (see block floating-point improved in Table 7.2).

We again refer to [Sche 05] for further details.

7.3.2 Filtering and Back-Projection

The performance of filtering and back-projection has been evaluated with the same datasets and with the same configurations which have already been used in the previous sections (see also Appendix B).

Table 7.3 shows the reconstruction performance of a PCI-based *ImageProX* accelerator board. The comparison of the back-projection speed and the overall reconstruction speed reveals that the reconstruction performance of this platform is limited by the bandwidth of the PCI bus. In theory, the PCI-X bandwidth is twice as high as the PCI bandwidth such that a correspondingly higher overall performance will result as soon as the PCI-X implementation is used instead. All filtering computations are completely concealed behind the projection upload over the PCI-X bus.

Currently, it is only possible to upload and filter the projection images on-the-fly, since our implementation requires all projection images in order to compute the back-projection result. However, the back-projection computation using the *Image-ProX* accelerator is as fast that it takes less than five seconds to back-project each of the datasets that are given in Table 9.1. Compared to the other considered hardware architectures the *ImageProX* accelerator thus delivers the fastest back-projection performance.

7.4 Summary

In this section we have developed a bit-accurate simulation framework for the filtering step. Furthermore, we have presented results for fixed-point convolution-based filtering, employing various scaling approaches and bit widths in the different computation stages. Our simulations include different scaling strategies for both the FFT computations as well as the intermediate processing steps of the convolution chain. Finally, we have shown a suitable configuration for the FPGA-based filtering implementation. This has also been our main contribution to the final FPGA-based FDK implementation on the ImageProX board which has been done at Siemens Healthcare.

Furthermore, we have briefly outlined and evaluated the mentioned FPGA-based implementation on the ImageProX accelerator. Although on-the-fly reconstruction is not supported, the accelerator board provides extremely fast back-projection processing thus being able to present the final reconstruction result to the physician nearly in real-time. A downside of the accelerator board is its PCI-based host connection, which results in significantly reduced overall reconstruction performance when compared to its back-projection processing speed.

Chapter 8

Performance Optimization of Selected Feldkamp Alternatives

Although many CT systems use the FDK method to solve the 3-D image reconstruction task, it is not without its short-comings. Therefore, we have described in Section 2.3 two alternative approaches: the theoretically exact and stable M-line method applied to a short-scan circle-plus-arc acquisition (Section 2.3.1) and the simultaneous algebraic reconstruction technique as a representative of the iterative approaches (Section 2.3.2).

While a thorough evaluation on several hardware platforms has been out of scope of this thesis, we evaluate in this chapter each of these techniques on an acceleration device that is – in our opinion – particularly well suited for a high performance implementation of the respective algorithm. In the following section we develop a highly optimized CBEA-based implementation of the M-line method. Section 8.2 then presents a CUDA-based implementation of the most time-consuming processing steps of iterative reconstruction approaches; the forward- and the back-projection.

We have chosen the CBEA for the M-line method because the CBEA provides comprehensive control in programming its processing cores, which may be a big advantage for the processing of the additional filtering steps. On the other hand GPUs may be the ideal candidates to implement the forward-projection step due to their texture units, which provide hardwired interpolation in the voxel volume. The performance evaluation of the M-line method on the CBEA has been presented at at the International Meeting on Fully Three-Dimensional Image Reconstruction in Radiology and Nuclear Medicine 2007 [Sche 07a], and our CUDA-accelerated forward- and back-projection module has been presented at the International Workshop on New Frontiers in High-performance and Hardware-aware Computing 2008 [Wein 08] and at the IEEE Nuclear Science Symposium and Medical Imaging Conference 2009 [Keck 09a].

8.1 M-line Method

In order to enable theoretically exact and stable FBP reconstruction in standard clinical scenarios we implemented a highly performance optimized version of the M-line method on the CBEA. Our software framework allows to compute the filtering and back-projection in parallel to the data acquisition, making it possible to deliver an on-the-fly-reconstruction.

In the following we consider the parallelized implementation and optimization of the M-line method and we demonstrate for the first time an on-the-fly-reconstruction while projection data are acquired. Our implementation supports the case of a non-ideal data acquisition and can thus reconstruct datasets from real C-arm CT scanners. We also compare the achieved results with our optimized CBEA implementation of the FDK method, which has been presented in Section 4.

8.1.1   Implementation

We implemented the basic processing chain of the M-line algorithm as a pipeline consisting of dedicated stages. One pipeline stage is responsible for loading the projections from the hard disk or over the network. As soon as a projection is available it can be processed by the subsequent pipeline stages. Our software framework extremely simplifies the implementation of such a pipeline. All pipeline stages are executed in parallel enabling on-the-fly-reconstructions in real-time.

The processing elements of the Cell processor are utilized by dispatching the associated parallel processing of a pipeline stage to a configurable number of SPEs. The PPE acts as the dispatcher which divides the processing of the considered pipeline stage into smaller tasks and assigns them to the available processing units. To minimize the control overhead we assign rather large tasks to the processing elements that further have to be divided into smaller tasks by the processing elements themselves. We take special care to hide any communication latencies via double buffering techniques during the dispatching and computation process.

The only downside of our approach is that similar to our FDK implementation the mapping of the available SPEs onto the pipeline stages is currently done statically. This means that we have to decide up front how many SPEs shall be used in each pipeline stage before program execution. Assigning each filtering step (F1 to F6) to a separate pipeline stage and thus to at least one SPE would result in a poor utilization of the SPEs only, which is a waste of computation resources. Technically, we compiled all filtering steps into one pipeline stage and one associated SPE program in order to circumvent this problem. The dispatching PPE identifies each filtering task via a special tag such that a filtering SPE can easily decide which processing task should be executed. Fortunately, together with necessary data buffers the complete SPE program fits into the Local Store, if temporary data buffers are shared among the different filtering task implementations. The PPE-side dispatching facility of the filtering pipeline stage takes care of synchronization and load-balancing between the individual filtering steps. Because of Local Store size restrictions, the filtering and back-projection tasks, however, had to be separated into two different pipeline stages and thus also into two different SPE programs.

An efficient implementation on the CBEA further requires to choose a proper parallelization strategy for each part of the algorithm that can deal with the limited Local Store size.

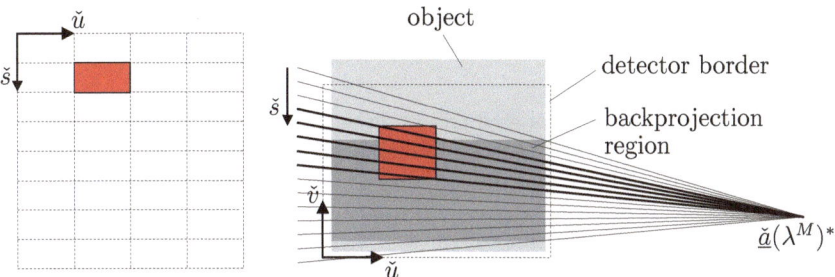

Figure 8.1: Implementation approach of forward rebinning. The colored box of the rebinned filtering lines (left) corresponds to the bold filtering lines in the colored box of the projection (right). It is only required to rebin filtering lines going through the back-projection region (see F6 for a definition).

F1 and F2 - Derivative and Cosine Weighting. The derivative computation is implemented in a row-based manner. Several rows of the resulting derived projection are assigned to an SPE at the same time. The SPE itself transfers the required rows of each involved projection (our current approximation of the derivative requires the considered projection together with the previous and next projection) to its Local Store, before performing the actual computations. Because the required computations for the derivative and the cosine weighting share a common factor we could easily combine the involved computations in order to achieve more efficiency.

F3 - Forward Rebinning. The rebinning computations could not be implemented in a line-based manner due to the limited size of the Local Store. An efficient parallelization strategy must further take into account that optimal sizes for memory transfers on the Cell processor are multiples of 128 bytes (32 single precision floating point values). We therefore decided to partition the rebinned image into blocks of 32×32 values. For each block the corresponding maximum shadow in the projection image is obtained by applying the rebinning equation to the four border values of a block (see Figure 8.1). Then we clip the resulting shadow with the detector boundary and transfer the associated data from main memory to the Local Store. After that the rebinning computations can be applied on the chosen partition and the resulting values can be transferred back to main memory. In order to avoid communication overhead we let the dispatching PPE assign several blocks to one SPE at the same time. The results are saved to a temporary buffer allocated in main memory.

F4 - Hilbert Filtering. The Hilbert filtering is implemented similar to the filtering step in the Feldkamp algorithm (see Section 4.2.1). The DFT of the spatial Hilbert kernel, however, does only have imaginary parts while the DFT of the spatial Ramp filter kernel, which is used in the FDK method, has only real parts. This required to slightly adapt the multiplication step in the frequency domain.

F5 - Backward Rebinning. The backward rebinning step is implemented using the parallelization strategy of the forward rebinning step, in reversed order.

F6 - π-Line Weighting. For each projection the associated π-line weighting mask $m(\lambda, u, v)$ has to be initialized, e.g. by loading it from the hard disk. In our current implementation we assumed that the hard disk is fast enough to load the mask images without introducing any time delays. While most of the mask values have the same value (1 or 0), a very simple compression scheme, e.g. based on run-length encoding would easily accelerate the hard disk transfers in a sufficient manner. The π-line weighting step itself is easily parallelized because it is nothing else than an element-wise multiplication of two 2D arrays.

Step 2 - Back-Projection. In our implementation of the back-projection for the FDK reconstruction method we were able to avoid detector boundary checks by restricting the processing only to volume voxels that are inside the FOV, thus always projecting onto the detector within its boundary. In order to account for that during the back-projection processing of the arc segments as well, we added detector boundary checks, because on the arc segments even voxels within the FOV may project to the outside of the detector.

8.1.2 Results

We evaluated the performance of our implementation using the same Cell-based Blade server board as we used in the evaluation of the FDK implementation. The board comprises two Cell processors running at 3.2 GHz each as well as 1 GB of main memory split across the two chips. The execution time of our M-line implementation was measured using a dataset consisting of 600 projection images of 1024×1024 pixels each. The number of projection images were 500 on the short-scan circle, 50 on the upper arc segment and also 50 on the lower arc segment. The average number of filtering lines per projection image was 1071. To achieve computation times that are not affected by FOV handling strategies we back-projected the cone-beam projections under consideration into a volume that fitted completely inside the FOV. Therefore, we used a volume consisting of $512 \times 512 \times 352$ voxels with a voxel size of 0.31^3 mm^3. During our measurements we removed any outliers by taking only the best runtime out of five measurements. After the correctness of the implementation was verified, we performed the measurements without doing the I/O transfers for loading the projection and mask images from the hard disk or over the network. This was necessary in order to achieve runtime measurements that were not affected by I/O bandwidth limitations of our current Cell Blade evaluation system.

In order to measure the execution times of each filtering step separately, we instrumented our code with SPE decrementer statements (performance counter on SPE side). Table 8.1 lists the execution time for filtering all 600 acquired projection images of the complete acquisition using one SPE. We took special care to avoid the influence from any other workload. The Hilbert filtering accounts for more than 33 % of the overall filtering computations. Compared to the filtering of our Cell-based FDK im-

Processing task	Time [s]	Percentage [%]
Derivative/Cosine Weighting	6.40	21.5
Forward rebinning	6.64	22.3
Hilbert Filtering	10.00	33.7
Backward rebinning	5.88	19.8
π-weighting	0.79	2.7
Total	29.71	100.00

Table 8.1: Performance results of all filtering stages within the M-line approach using one SPE.

	Number of SPEs (filtering/back-projection)						
	using one Cell processor			using two Cell processors			
	1/7	2/6	3/5	1/15	2/14	3/13	4/12
M-line (short-scan circle plus two arc segments)							
Time [s]	33.25	**30.05**	35.24	31.20	17.38	**14.64**	15.61
pps	18.05	**20.00**	17.03	19.23	34.52	**40.98**	38.44
fps	10.59	**11.71**	9.99	11.28	20.25	**24.04**	22.55
FDK (short-scan circle only)							
Time [s]	**19.80**	22.99	27.52	**9.43**	10.07	10.81	
pps	**25.15**	21.66	18.10	**52.81**	49.45	46.07	
fps	**17.78**	15.31	12.79	**37.33**	34.96	32.56	

Table 8.2: Overall pipelined execution of the filtering and back-projection for the M-line method and the FDK method.

plementation (see Section 4.2) the computing time of filtering[1] increases by a factor of 3.5 in the exact approach. Due to the random memory accesses during forward and backward rebinning, the corresponding computations are the most expensive ones. Usually there are more filtering lines than rows in the projection images. Because of this reason the forward rebinning accounts for more processing time in comparison to the backward rebinning,

During the validation of the performance of the overall pipeline execution (simultaneous, parallel execution of filtering and back-projection in a pipeline) we used the "gettimeofday" function on the PPE. This ensures that all overhead during program execution (e.g., starting the SPE threads) are included in the measurements.

Table 8.2 shows the achieved results for various configurations of used SPEs for filtering and back-projection, respectively. For comparison purposes we also computed FDK reconstructions with the same SPE configuration using only the projection images from the short-scan circle. We also give the numbers of projection images that can be processed per second (pps). This number is important because on-the-fly-reconstruction can only be achieved when the reconstruction system is able to process at least the same number of projections per second than the scanning de-

---

[1]This includes all M-line filtering steps F1 to F6.

vice can deliver. Recent C-arm devices achieve rates of 30 pps for 1k images. For convenience, we also calculated the number of 512×512 image slices, that can be reconstructed in one second (frames per second, fps) as this number is often used in research for comparison purposes. One can see that, in contrast to the FDK method, the reconstruction speed of the M-line method is limited by the processing time of the SPEs used for the filtering pipeline stage. Using only one Cell processor of our dual Cell Blade two filtering SPEs and using both Cell processors even three filtering SPEs are required in order to achieve optimal performance. Otherwise the execution time is limited either by the filtering performance or by the back-projection performance. The back-projection performance is roughly comparable to the one used in the FDK implementation. Both reconstruction approaches, however, achieve on-the-fly-reconstruction using two Cell processors.

8.2 Iterative Reconstruction

In Section 6 we focused on an efficient GPU implementation of the Feldkamp algorithm. The most time-consuming part of that method is the back-projection step. As described in Section 2.3.2 iterative reconstruction algorithms require another very compute-intensive processing step additionally to the back-projection: the forward-projection through the voxel-volume.

In the following we present an efficient GPU implementation of forward-projection based on ray casting. Ray casting is a well-known method in volume rendering and it can be efficiently implemented by using the texture hardware of modern GPUs [Enge 06].

First, we explain the basic structure of ray casting. We further describe all important details of an efficient GPU-based implementation of ray casting and evaluate its performance. Finally we estimate the achievable computational performance of SART using GPUs based on our performance evaluation of back-projection and forward-projection.

8.2.1 Basic Structure of Ray Casting

The basic idea of ray casting is to directly evaluate the line integrals of the object density function according to Equation (2.1) along rays that are traversed from the position of the X-ray camera to the detector plane. Neglecting possible supersampling on the detector plane for each sample position on the detector a single ray is cast into the volume. Then the volume data is resampled at discrete positions along the ray. Figure 8.2 illustrates the principle of ray casting. Algorithm 7 details the algorithmic steps, which are executed during each forward-projection step.

Accordingly, forward-projection based on ray casting can be split into the following components:

Ray Initialization. For each pixel position $(\check{u}, \check{v})^T$ on the detector plane of the considered projection this component sets up a ray, which emerges from the

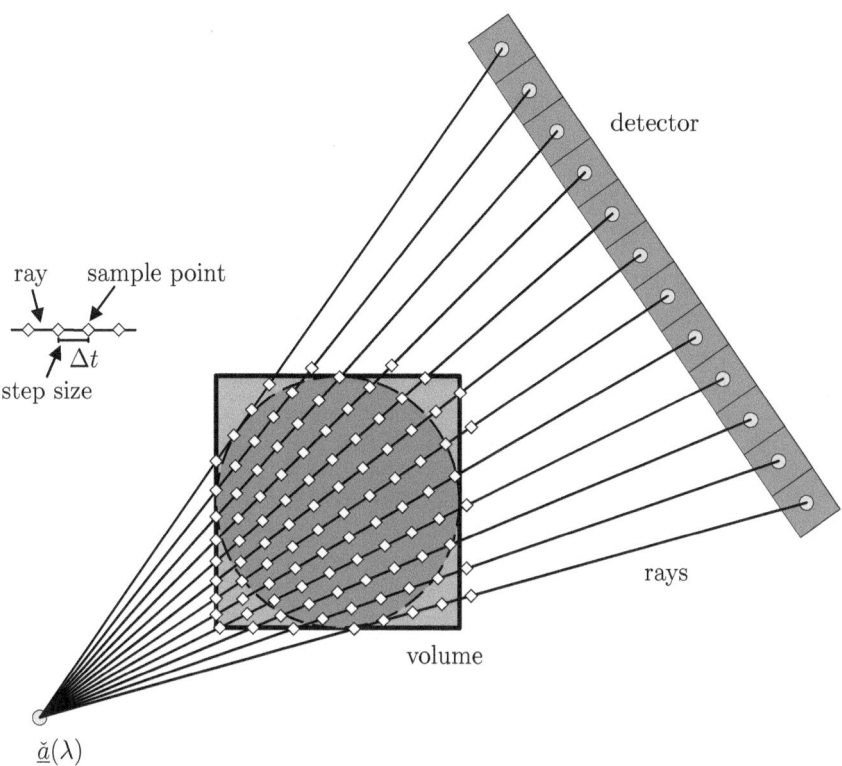

Figure 8.2: Ray casting principle. For each detector element one ray is traced. The ray is sampled at discrete positions in the volume to evaluate the line integrals. The sampling interval on the ray is denoted by Δt. The X-ray source position is indicated by $\underline{\breve{a}}(\lambda)$ expressed in voxel coordinates.

corresponding source position $\underline{\breve{a}}(\lambda) = (\breve{a}_x, \breve{a}_y, \breve{a}_z)^T$ of the X-ray camera[2]. We use a parametric representation of the ray. The ray is therefore defined by

$$\underline{\breve{x}} = (\breve{x}, \breve{y}, \breve{z})^T = \underline{\breve{a}}(\lambda) + t\underline{\breve{\theta}}(\breve{u}, \breve{v}), \qquad (8.1)$$

where $t \in \mathbb{R}$ is a parameter indicating the extent of the ray from $\underline{\breve{a}}(\lambda)$ and $\underline{\breve{\theta}}(\breve{u}, \breve{v}) = (\breve{\theta}_x, \breve{\theta}_y, \breve{\theta}_z)^T$ specifies the direction of the ray. The vectors $\underline{\breve{x}}$, $\underline{\breve{a}}(\lambda)$, and $\underline{\breve{\theta}}(\breve{u}, \breve{v})$ are expressed in voxel coordinates and the vector $(\breve{u}, \breve{v})^T$ is expressed in pixel coordinates.

Let $\check{\mathbf{P}}(\lambda)$ be the corresponding projection matrix, which projects a point expressed in voxel coordinates to a detector position expressed in pixel coordi-

---

[2] In the case of an ideal circular acquisition the source position $\underline{a}(\lambda)$ (in world coordinates) at rotation angle λ is defined by Equation (2.3).

Algorithm 7: Pseudo-code for forward-projection based on ray casting.

Input: projection matrix $\check{\mathbf{P}}$
Input: step size Δt along ray
Input: volume data $\check{\mathbf{V}}$
Result: projection $\check{\mathbf{I}}$

1 Extract source position from $\check{\mathbf{P}}$;
2 **foreach** *ray* $(\check{u}, \check{v})^T$ *of projection* $\check{\mathbf{I}}$ **do**
3 | $\check{\mathbf{I}}[\check{u}, \check{v}] = 0$;
4 | Extract ray direction from $\check{\mathbf{P}}$;
5 | Compute volume entry and exit position;
6 | **while** *ray position in volume* **do**
7 | | Access data value at current position from $\check{\mathbf{V}}$;
8 | | Multiply data value with the step size Δt and accumulate it to $\check{\mathbf{I}}[\check{u}, \check{v}]$;
9 | | Advance position along ray according to step size Δt;
10 | **end**
11 | Rescale $\check{\mathbf{I}}[\check{u}, \check{v}]$ to world coordinate system units;
12 **end**

---

nates[3]. Then the source position vector $\underline{\check{a}}(\lambda)$ (in voxel coordinates) is given by [Gali 03]

$$\underline{\check{a}}(\lambda) = -\check{\mathbf{P}}(\lambda)[:, 0:2]^{-1}\check{\mathbf{P}}(\lambda)[:, 3], \qquad (8.2)$$

where $\check{\mathbf{P}}(\lambda)[:, 0:2]$ refers to the matrix containing the first three columns of $\check{\mathbf{P}}(\lambda)$ and $\check{\mathbf{P}}(\lambda)[:, 3]$ represents the fourth column of $\check{\mathbf{P}}(\lambda)$. It is also possible to determine the direction $\underline{\check{\theta}}(\check{u}, \check{v})$ without an explicit knowledge of the three-dimensional coordinates of the detector pixel $(\check{u}, \check{v})^T$. The resulting direction vector is given by [Gali 03]

$$\underline{\check{\theta}}(\check{u}, \check{v}) = -\check{\mathbf{P}}(\lambda)[:, 0:2]^{-1}(\check{u}, \check{v}, 1)^T. \qquad (8.3)$$

In the following we assume that the ray direction has been normalized according to $||\underline{\check{\theta}}(\check{u}, \check{v})||_2 = 1$.

The ray set up further includes the computation of the volume entry and exit position defined as the first and last intersection of the ray with the bounding geometry of the volume dataset.

Traversal Loop. In order to evaluate the line integral the main component traverses along the ray and samples it at discrete positions. The traversal loop then scans the ray at these positions. In each iteration of the loop the following subcomponents are executed.

---

[3]In the case of an ideal circular acquisition the projection matrix $\check{\mathbf{P}}(\lambda)$ at rotation angle λ is given by Equation (2.16).

Data Access. The volume dataset is accessed at the current ray position and the corresponding value is interpolated from the discrete volume data using for example trilinear interpolation. Finally, the resulting value is accumulated to the current line integral value of that ray.

Advance Ray Position. The current ray position is advanced to the next sampling position along the ray. Rays are sampled uniformly. Therefore the next sampling position is defined by

$$\check{x} = \check{a}(\lambda) + (t + \Delta t)\check{\theta}(\check{u}, \check{v}),\tag{8.4}$$

where Δt defines the step size and t determines the current ray position.

Ray Termination. This subcomponent exits the traversal loop when the ray leaves the volume.

Rescale ray sum. Ray casting as described above approximates the forward-projection that is given by the term

$$\sum_{j=0}^{J-1} a_{mj,n}\hat{x}_j^{k+1,n-1}\tag{8.5}$$

of Equation (2.51). Here, the matrix entries $a_{mj,n}$ are expressed in units of the world coordinate system. The computations of the traversal loop, however, have been done in voxel coordinates. It is therefore necessary to rescale the computed ray sum to world coordinates.

In order to rescale the ray sum we first express the direction vector $\underline{\theta}(\check{u}, \check{v}) = (\check{\theta}_x, \check{\theta}_y, \check{\theta}_z)^T$ of Equation (8.1) with respect to the world coordinate system:

$$\underline{\theta}(u, v) = \begin{pmatrix} \theta_x(u, v) \\ \theta_y(u, v) \\ \theta_z(u, v) \end{pmatrix} = \begin{pmatrix} dx & 0 & 0 \\ 0 & dy & 0 \\ 0 & 0 & dz \end{pmatrix} \cdot \underline{\check{\theta}}(\check{u}, \check{v}) = \begin{pmatrix} dx \cdot \check{\theta}_x(\check{u}, \check{v}) \\ dy \cdot \check{\theta}_y(\check{u}, \check{v}) \\ dz \cdot \check{\theta}_z(\check{u}, \check{v}) \end{pmatrix}.$$
$$\tag{8.6}$$

The computed ray sum thus has to be rescaled by multiplying it with the factor

$$n_f = \frac{||\underline{\theta}(u, v)||_2}{||\underline{\check{\theta}}(\check{u}, \check{v})||_2}\tag{8.7}$$

$$= \sqrt{(dx \cdot \check{\theta}_x(\check{u}, \check{v}))^2 + (dy \cdot \check{\theta}_y(\check{u}, \check{v}))^2 + (dz \cdot \check{\theta}_z(\check{u}, \check{v}))^2}.\tag{8.8}$$

Note that $\underline{\check{\theta}}(\check{u}, \check{v})$ has been normalized during ray set-up and thus $||\underline{\check{\theta}}(\check{u}, \check{v})||_2 = 1$.

The following section describes how the different components of ray casting as described above can be implemented on GPUs using CUDA.

8.2.2 Implementation of Ray Casting

During ray casting the rays can be processed independently of each other. This parallelism is compatible with hardware parallelism in GPUs: the operations of a single ray are associated with a single thread of the kernel program, which is responsible

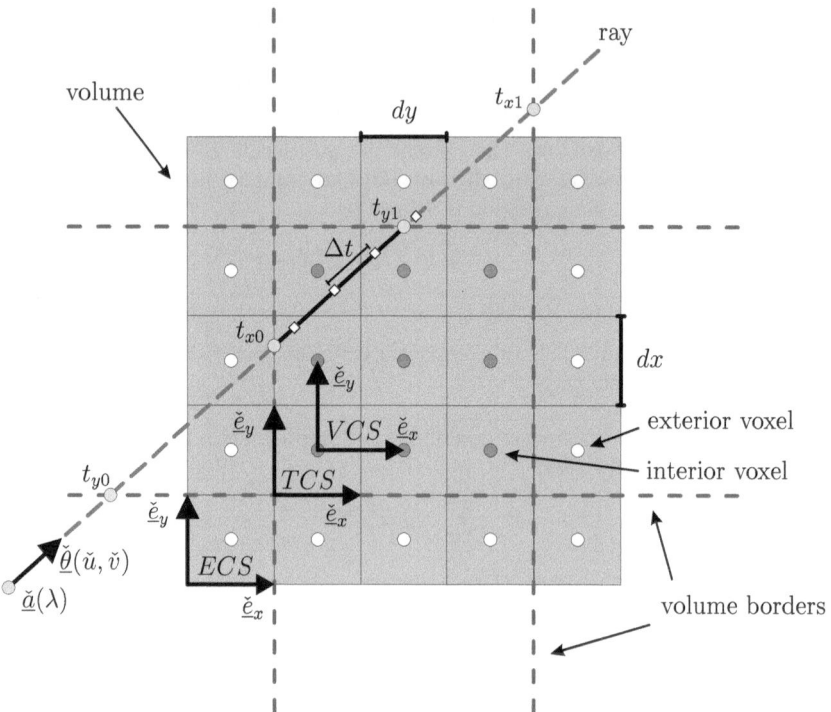

Figure 8.3: Detailed look at the ray casting implementation. Here, one ray is given by the source position $\breve{\underline{a}}(\lambda)$ and the direction vector $\breve{\underline{\theta}}(\breve{u}, \breve{v})$ pointing to the detector element $(\breve{u}, \breve{v})^T$.

to compute the line integrals of a projection. Additionally, the volume data is stored in a three-dimensional texture object, and is thus accessed with the high internal memory bandwidth of a GPU and hardware-accelerated trilinear interpolation.

The computations during the processing of a ray are performed with respect to the voxel coordinate system (VCS). The VCS is a right-handed coordinate system, it is aligned to the center of voxel $(0, 0, 0)^T$ and the voxel size is normalized to 1 in each direction (see Figure 8.3). Textures in CUDA[4], however, are defined with respect to a different coordinate system that is aligned to the boundary of the volume. In the following we refer to this coordinate system as the texture coordinate system (TCS).

---

[4] We only use unnormalized textures in CUDA. Unnormalized textures are referenced using floating-point coordinates in the range $[0, N)$ where N is the size of the texture in the dimension corresponding to the coordinate. For example, a texture that is 64×32 in size will be referenced with coordinates in the range $[0, 63]$ and $[0, 31]$ for the first and second dimension, respectively. See [NVID 09] for more details.

The following transform comprises the necessary translation of homogeneous texture coordinates to the VCS:

$$\mathbf{T}_{TCS} = \begin{bmatrix} 1 & 0 & 0 & -0.5 \\ 0 & 1 & 0 & -0.5 \\ 0 & 0 & 1 & -0.5 \\ 0 & 0 & 0 & 1 \end{bmatrix} \tag{8.9}$$

Furthermore, boundary accesses to the texture have to be treated specially in order to compute an accurate ray sum at the border of the volume. For example the ray sum is not computed correctly for the last two sampling points on the ray in Figure 8.3. The texture coordinates are simply clamped[5] to the border of the texture and the wrong points are sampled. In order to ensure a correct sampling at the border of the volume we enlarge the texture by adding border voxels (exterior voxels) around the texture and initializing them with the value 0. Otherwise texture accesses at the border region would be clamped to the wrong volume location. The enhanced texture defines another coordinate system: the extended texture coordinate system (ECS). The following transform comprises the translation of enhanced texture coordinates in homogeneous representation to the coordinates of the TCS:

$$\mathbf{T}_{ECS} = \begin{bmatrix} 1 & 0 & 0 & -1.0 \\ 0 & 1 & 0 & -1.0 \\ 0 & 0 & 1 & -1.0 \\ 0 & 0 & 0 & 1 \end{bmatrix} \tag{8.10}$$

In order to compute all processing steps of the ray casting algorithm within the ECS each projection matrix $\check{\mathbf{P}}(\lambda)$ is modified during ray initialization according to

$$\check{\mathbf{P}}(\lambda) \cdot \mathbf{T}_{TCS} \cdot \mathbf{T}_{ECS} \tag{8.11}$$

before kernel execution. This approach improves the efficiency of our implementation because all computations regarding the correct handling of the coordinate systems are moved out of the traversal loop.

We further compute $\check{\mathbf{P}}(\lambda)[:,0:2]^{-1}$ and $\underline{\check{a}}(\lambda)$ and copy their corresponding entries to constant device memory. Then the ray casting kernel is started launching a single thread for each sample position on the detector. It facilitates all components mentioned in the previous section: the remaining steps of ray initialization (computation of ray direction, entry, and exit position), ray traversal, data access, ray termination, and ray normalization.

---

[5] Textures in CUDA can be accessed using different addressing modes. The addressing mode defines what happens when texture coordinates are out of range. In CUDA version 2.3 only the "clamped" addressing mode is available for unnormalized textures: Let N be the size of the texture in the dimension corresponding to the considered coordinate. Coordinates that are outside the range $[0, N)$ are clamped. Values below 0 are set to 0 and values greater or equal to N are set to $N - 1$. See [NVID 09] for more details.

In order to compute the entry and exit positions we follow the approach in [Sidd 85]. First, Equation (8.4) is solved for t and all parameter values of t are computed where the ray intersects with one of the sides of the volume cube[6]:

$$
\begin{aligned}
t_{x0} &= \frac{1 - \breve{a}_x}{\breve{\theta}_x}, & t_{x1} &= \frac{(N_x + 1) - \breve{a}_x}{\breve{\theta}_x}, \\
t_{y0} &= \frac{1 - \breve{a}_y}{\breve{\theta}_y}, & t_{y1} &= \frac{(N_y + 1) - \breve{a}_y}{\breve{\theta}_y}, \\
t_{z0} &= \frac{1 - \breve{a}_z}{\breve{\theta}_z}, & t_{z1} &= \frac{(N_z + 1) - \breve{a}_z}{\breve{\theta}_z}.
\end{aligned}
\tag{8.12}
$$

Here, the number of voxels in the volume (excluding the exterior voxels) is given by $N_x \times N_y \times N_z$.

If the denominator is zero in one of these equations, then the ray is parallel to the volume side under consideration and the result is undefined. In such a case we simply exclude the corresponding equation from the following computations.

In terms of the parametric values given by Equation (8.12) the entry and exit positions $t_{\min}$ and $t_{\max}$, respectively, are computed by

$$
\begin{aligned}
t_{\min} &= \max\left(\min(t_{x0}, t_{x1}), \min(t_{y0}, t_{y1}), \min(t_{z0}, t_{z1})\right), & (8.13) \\
t_{\max} &= \min\left(\max(t_{x0}, t_{x1}), \max(t_{y0}, t_{y1}), \max(t_{z0}, t_{z1})\right), & (8.14)
\end{aligned}
$$

where the functions "min" and "max" select the minimum and maximum value of their argument list, respectively. The ray does only intersect the volume cube if $t_{\min}$ is less than $t_{\max}$. Figure 8.3 illustrates the computed values for a single ray, where the final values of $t_{\min}$ and $t_{\max}$ are given by t_{x0} and t_{y1}, respectively.

The traversal loop then computes the normalized ray sum according to Algorithm 8. The CUDA-function "tex3D" accesses a texture at the specified coordinates. The texture has been configured to use trilinear interpolation. The last sample position may be already outside of the volume cube but it must be treated specially in order to add to the ray sum also the remaining fraction of Δt for that sample position.

In volume rendering applications the performance of ray casting can be improved by additional acceleration methods. For example, early ray termination, adaptive sampling, and empty-space skipping can be used to significantly improve the rendering performance [Enge 06]. It is, however, very problematic to apply these acceleration techniques in the context of iterative cone-beam reconstruction. In this domain, the line integrals have to be computed as accurately as possible. Moreover, the attenuation coefficients are updated frequently, which does not justify to apply expensive volume preprocessing methods during the reconstruction process.

8.2.3   Results

In order to evaluate the ray casting performance of our GPU implementation, we used again the same workstation (*Intel Xeon* Quad-core processor (E5440) running

---

[6]The volume cube consists only of the interior voxels (see Figure 8.3).

Algorithm 8: Pseudo-code of the traversal loop in the kernel program of ray casting

---

Input: pixel position $(\check{u}, \check{v})^T$
Input: step size Δt along ray
Input: source position $\underline{\check{a}} = (\check{a}_x, \check{a}_y, \check{a}_z)^T$
Input: ray direction $\underline{\check{\theta}} = (\check{\theta}_x, \check{\theta}_y, \check{\theta}_z)^T$
Input: entry position $t_{\min}$ and exit position $t_{\max}$
Input: normalization factor n_f
Input: volume texture $\check{\mathbf{V}}$
Result: projection $\check{\mathbf{I}}$

1 float $t = t_{\min}$;
2 float $val = 0.0f$;
   // traversal loop
3 **while** $(t < t_{\max})$ **do**
4 $\quad$ float $\check{x} = \check{a}_x + t \cdot \check{\theta}_x$;
5 $\quad$ float $\check{y} = \check{a}_y + t \cdot \check{\theta}_y$;
6 $\quad$ float $\check{z} = \check{a}_z + t \cdot \check{\theta}_z$;
7 $\quad$ $val = val + \text{tex3D}(\check{\mathbf{V}}, \check{x}, \check{y}, \check{z})$;
8 $\quad$ $t = t + \Delta t$;
9 **end**
   // ray normalization
10 $val = val \cdot n_f$;
   // handle last sample point
11 **if** $((t - \frac{\Delta t}{2}) < t_{\max})$ **then**
12 $\quad$ float $\check{x} = \check{a}_x + t \cdot \check{\theta}_x$;
13 $\quad$ float $\check{y} = \check{a}_y + t \cdot \check{\theta}_y$;
14 $\quad$ float $\check{z} = \check{a}_z + t \cdot \check{\theta}_z$;
15 $\quad$ $val = val + (t - \frac{\Delta t}{2}) \cdot \frac{n_f}{\Delta t} \cdot \text{tex3D}(\check{\mathbf{V}}, \check{x}, \check{y}, \check{z})$;
16 **end**
   // save result
17 $\check{\mathbf{I}}[\check{u}, \check{v}] = val$;

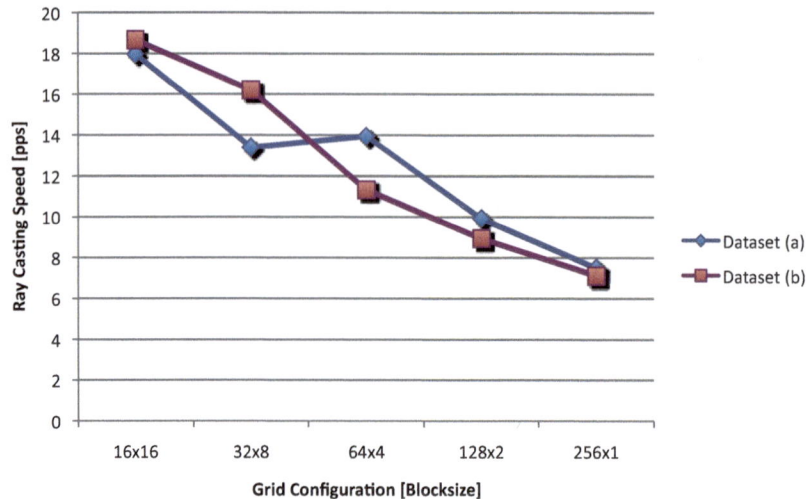

Figure 8.4: Ray casting performance for different grid configurations. The number of forward-projections that can be processed per second (pps) are given. During ray casting a step size of 1.0 of the voxel size has been used.

at 2.83 GHz) and installed the *Tesla C1060* accelerator from Nvidia. We computed forward-projections of the two real datasets that have already been used during the evaluation of the FDK method (see Appendix B for a detailed description of the datasets). For both datasets we used a volume that was reconstructed using the FDK method. The volume had a size of 512^3 voxels. The voxel size was chosen such that the complete FOV fits into the volume. It was configured to 0.38 mm for Dataset (a) and 0.46 mm for Dataset (b).

In order to load the volume into the 3-D texture array 0.26 seconds are required. The ray casting kernel compiled to 12 registers, which results in the maximum possible warp occupancy that is available on the used Tesla device. The shared memory usage did not limit the warp occupancy either.

In order to further tune the performance we executed the ray casting processing with different grid configurations. Figure 8.4 shows the results. It can be seen that it is important to improve data locality during the ray traversal loop. We observed the best performance using a grid configuration with a block size of 16 × 16 pixels. The geometry of the dataset also influences the access pattern during the ray traversal loop. Therefore, the curves in Figure 8.4 corresponding to the two datasets slightly vary from each other. In the following we kept the grid configuration fixed and used a block size of 16 × 16 pixels.

We further examined the influence of the step size on the performance of ray casting by executing our ray casting kernel with different step sizes. Table 8.3 shows the results for the two considered datasets. For Dataset (a) all 414 projections have been forward-projected and for Dataset (b) all 543 projections have been forward-

Stepsize [voxel units]	0.10	0.25	0.50	0.75	1.00
Dataset (a)					
Time [s]	212.25	86.62	44.45	30.03	23.03
pps	1.95	4.78	9.31	13.79	17.98
Dataset (b)					
Time [s]	282.54	113.38	57.18	38.38	29.08
pps	1.92	4.79	9.50	14.15	18.67

Table 8.3: GPU performance results of ray casting for the considered datasets using different step sizes.

	Dataset (a)		Dataset (b)	
Processing Step	Time [s]	pps	Time [s]	pps
Back-Projection	10.25	40.39	15.16	35.82
Forward-Projection	23.03	17.98	29.08	18.64
Texture Updates	38.83	10.66	50.93	10.66
One SART Iteration	>72.11	<5.74	>95.17	<5.71

Table 8.4: GPU performance results of the computationally most demanding processing steps of SART. All processing steps are executed on a Tesla C1060 device from Nvidia. The results are given for a single iteration. The step size during ray casting was 1.0.

projected. The volume texture was loaded only once and the projection results were not transferred to the host. As expected the achieved processing times nearly scale linearly with the configured step size. While smaller step sizes may improve the image quality of the overall reconstruction result, the computational performance is severely limited.

The forward-projection at a step size of 1.0 accounts for roughly twice as much processing time compared to the back-projection processing (see Table 8.4). Back-projection takes longer compared to the measurements in Section 6.3 because the increased voxel size causes more texture cache misses.

Using CUDA Version 2.3 it is not yet possible to share the volume memory between back-projection and forward-projection. The back-projection is implemented using global memory, which is linearly allocated, while the forward-projection accesses the volume memory via a 3-D texture. 3-D textures use a proprietary data layout that is optimized for access locality. It is thus required to allocate twice as much memory for the volume and after the back-projection of each projection image the 3-D texture has to be updated. Transferring the volume to the 3-D texture takes 0.1 seconds. It can be seen in Table 8.4 that the texture update dominates the overall execution time of SART. In contrast, SIRT updates the texture only once in each iteration. Likewise, the texture update time can be reduced by applying an ordered subset approach.

Ray casting is, however, not the only approach in order to compute the forward-projection step. Indeed, several different ways have been introduced in the literature.

A detailed comparison can be found in [Xu 06]. Due to the expensive texture updates, it might be beneficial to implement the forward-projection step using the Joseph method [Jose 83], which requires only 2-D texture accesses.

At the same time the volume could be saved to a pitched linear 2-D texture representation, which allows to share the memory of the volume with the back-projection. From a computational point of view this completely avoids the texture updates. Unfortunately, at the time we implemented the ray casting algorithm pitched linear textures was not available in CUDA.

8.3 Summary

We have developed a parallelized and highly optimized implementation of two alternative reconstruction approaches to the Feldkamp algorithm.

In particular, using the CBEA we have evaluated the computational performance of the M-line method, which is a representative of a theoretically exact and stable cone-beam reconstruction algorithm. In this regard, we have shown that the execution time of filtering increases only by a factor of 3.5 compared to the FDK method. We have demonstrated that with our dual Cell Blade an M-line reconstruction for a standard clinical scenario can be computed in 14.64 seconds (40.98 pps) using a short-scan circle plus two arcs acquisition. This leverages high quality cone-beam CT reconstructions on-the-fly, which means that all required computations are hidden behind the scan-time of the used X-ray device.

Finally, we have presented an efficient implementation of the computationally most demanding steps in iterative reconstruction algorithms on off-the-shelf graphics boards. Because the back-projection step can be implemented similar to the FDK method we have especially considered the forward-projection step. Our implementation is based on a ray casting algorithm in order to make efficient use of the texture hardware in current graphics accelerators. Using a reasonable parameter configuration the forward-projection step requires roughly twice as much processing time as the back-projection step. However, the necessary texture updates of the voxel volume between back-projection and forward-projection has been shown to be a huge bottleneck, which can only be reduced by applying an ordered subset approach or SIRT like iterative algorithms.

Chapter 9

Conclusions

This chapter summarizes the main contributions and results of this work and describes future directions for research in the field of hardware-accelerated cone-beam CT reconstruction.

9.1 Summary

We have presented both the design and the implementation of a software architecture that is well suited to implement and accelerate the computationally intensive task of 3-D reconstruction in CT imaging. Software engineering techniques play an important role in the overall design and can improve the efficiency, flexibility, and portability of the whole reconstruction system.

In this regard, the parallel reconstruction algorithms can be mapped to a design approach that combines the pipeline design pattern with the master/worker design pattern. We have illustrated how the design can act as a hardware abstraction layer on top of different acceleration architectures. It even allows to combine the use of several acceleration hardware platforms for different parts of the algorithm in a heterogeneous environment.

In order to evaluate the suitability of four different state-of-the-art hardware architectures for their usage in cone-beam CT reconstruction we have implemented highly optimized versions of the FDK method for each of these hardware architectures. Furthermore, we have evaluated their reconstruction performance using two medical datasets that were acquired using a standard C-arm device.

It is difficult – if not impossible – to objectively compare the reconstruction speed of different hardware architectures as long as not the same precondition is fulfilled. Linear scaling and comparison of published results may lead to wrong conclusions concerning the achievable reconstruction speed due to the use of different hardware, different datasets, different reconstruction parameters, and due to many implementations that assume an ideal geometric acquisition, which is unfortunately not the case in most practical cone-beam CT scanners.

Table 9.1 shows a comparison of the achievable reconstruction speed for the FDK method using the hardware architectures that have been discussed in this thesis. All measurements have been done using the same reconstruction parameters and using the same two medical datasets. In order that an FDK reconstruction can be computed

Hardware	Filtering		Back-Projection		Overall	
	[s]	pps	[s]	pps	[s]	pps
Dataset (a), convolution length 2048						
CPU (Intel quad-core, 2.3 GHz)	3.5	118.8	138.0	3.0	140.0	3.0
Cell processor (8 SPEs, 3.2 GHz)	0.8	503.0	21.0	19.7	24.0	17.2
GPU (Nvidia Tesla C1060)	1.3	309.0	5.2	79.3	7.3	57.1
FPGA (*ImageProX*)			3.9	107.3	11.2	36.9
Dataset (b), convolution length 4096						
CPU (Intel quad-core, 2.3 GHz)	5.6	97.9	182.0	3.0	186.0	2.9
Cell processor (8 SPEs, 3.2 GHz)	1.9	287.5	27.7	19.6	31.9	17.0
GPU (Nvidia Tesla C1060)	3.5	156.5	8.2	66.1	12.6	43.1
FPGA (*ImageProX*)			4.4	124.5	15.0	36.3

Table 9.1: Reconstruction performance results of the FDK method (filtering and back-projection) for all hardware alternatives under consideration.

on-the-fly using a current practical cone-beam CT scanner, at least 30 projections per second must be processed. It can be seen from Table 9.1 that current GPU devices are ideal candidates when reconstructions shall be computed on-the-fly while projection data is being acquired.

An on-the-fly reconstruction can also be achieved when using two Cell processors. It is, however, difficult to find commercial solutions that offer two Cell processors on a single mainboard. As far as we know, currently only Cell Blades exist on the market that provide two Cell processors acting as an SMP[1] machine.

Using the *ImageProX* FPGA board it is only possible to upload and filter the projection images on-the-fly, since our implementation requires all projection images in order to compute the back-projection result. However, the back-projection computation using the *ImageProX* accelerator is as fast that it takes less than five seconds to back-project each of the datasets that are given in Table 9.1. Compared to the other considered hardware architectures the *ImageProX* accelerator delivers the fastest back-projection performance.

On the other hand, it is nearly impossible to build systems that are able to accomplish on-the-fly reconstructions using only a few cores of current general-purpose processors (e.g., Intel- or AMD-based). Their reconstruction performance is far away from the speed that is exhibited by the more specialized architectures under consideration. The achieved results demonstrate that a performance increase of an order of magnitude and even more is achievable compared to recent high performance general-purpose computing platforms (see again Table 9.1).

High-end graphics accelerators currently deliver the fastest overall reconstruction speeds. The processing power of high-end GPU devices delivers the compute power to process more than 40 projections per second. Concerning real-time imaging, the achieved performance of the FDK method thus shows that there are still compu-

---

[1] Symmetric Multiprocessing (SMP)

tational resources available to compute further preprocessing tasks such as beam hardening correction, truncation correction, or scatter correction, for instance.

While implementation complexity typically tends to be comparatively low for CPU-based systems, highly optimized CPU implementations are getting as complicated as implementations for more specialized architectures. This is especially true for Cell processor based systems and FPGA accelerators. According to our experience, GPU systems provide a reasonable balance between implementation effort and achievable reconstruction speed.

A downside of the GPUs is their co-processor based architecture. A corresponding CPU core has to be present in order to control and to synchronize the GPU calculations. We observed high load on the CPU during GPU computations indicating that synchronization is presently still being accomplished using busy-waiting loops. In a quad-core Intel system, we could only compute on seven hyper-threads without affecting the GPU reconstruction speed significantly. Since we have not used the asynchronous API[2] functions and the streaming programming interface of CUDA yet, we expect that it will be possible to reduce the load on the host system that is caused by GPU calculations. The use of this programming API will further enable to hide the time needed for data uploads to the GPU behind actual GPU computations, which will improve reconstruction speed even more.

Although many CT systems use the FDK method to solve the 3-D image reconstruction task, it is not without its short-comings. Therefore, we have described two alternative approaches: the theoretically exact and stable M-line method applied to a short-scan circle-plus-arc acquisition and the simultaneous algebraic reconstruction technique as a representative of the iterative approaches. While a thorough evaluation on several hardware platforms has been out of scope of this thesis, each of these techniques has been evaluated on an acceleration device that is – in our opinion – particularly well suited for a high performance implementation of the respective algorithm.

The M-line method totally resolves the problem of cone artifacts, which result from the approximative nature of the state-of-the-art FDK method. Therefore, small object details may be covered complicating their distinction. At the same time, the M-line method can be implemented in the efficient FBP framework. We presented a performance optimized implementation of the M-line method on the CBEA for a circular short-scan plus arc acquisition. Our implementation further respects the non-ideal acquisition geometry of practical C-arm systems. Compared to the FDK method the computing time of the filtering steps of the M-line method increased by a factor of three. Using two Cell processors the CBEA still offered enough computational resources to compute the reconstruction on-the-fly, but an additional SPE was necessary for the computations of the filtering steps.

Iterative reconstruction methods provide an entirely different way to solve the CT reconstruction task and, in certain situations, they achieve a better image quality compared to that of the FDK method or even the M-line method. For example this is the case when a sufficiently large number of projections is not feasible or simply not desired to measure. Iterative approaches have also the opportunity to achieve better image quality when the projections are not uniformly distributed over the scan

---

[2] Application programming interface (API)

trajectory. The two computationally most expensive steps are the back-projection and the forward-projection. We have examined an optimized implementation of both steps on a high-performance GPU device. The implementation of the back-projection step has been done in the FDK method. For the forward-projection step we used a ray casting algorithm, which can be ideally mapped to the texture hardware of current GPUs. The forward-projection accounts at least for twice as much processing time as the back-projection. Using the GPUs as acceleration hardware it becomes feasible to use iterative methods for certain applications in practical cone-beam reconstruction devices but still at the cost of highly increased computation times.

We conclude that especially in flat-panel cone-beam CT (e.g., C-arm devices) the Cell chip, graphics boards, and FPGA-based platforms represent very promising computing architectures. In particular, both the Cell processor and GPU hardware provide the possibility to be programmed rather elegantly in a high level programming language. This feature can significantly contribute to reduce the innovation cycles of the reconstruction system in practical scanning devices.

9.2 Future Work

Although we provided a comprehensive overview of the field of hardware-accelerated cone-beam CT reconstruction there are some topics that have not been evaluated in this thesis but are worth being investigated in the future. In the following we will discuss the most promising topics.

There are other computing platforms that have not been considered in this thesis. Intel, for example, is doing research on a hybrid between a multi-core CPU and a GPU. Its codename was Larrabee. Like CPUs the Larrabee chip has a coherent cache hierarchy and is compatible to the x86 architecture. But it has also GPU-like features such as its wide SIMD vector units and its texture sampling hardware.

In this thesis we considered only graphics cards from Nvidia. Other GPUs, e.g. from AMD/ATI, could be applied to cone-beam CT reconstruction as well. These GPUs, however, do not support CUDA and thus have to be programmed in a different way.

Recently, an open programming standard emerged for general purpose computing on heterogeneous systems. It is called the Open Computing Language (OpenCL). Several vendors already support OpenCL for their computing hardware. For example, Nvidia, AMD/ATI, and IBM have already released an SDK enabling OpenCL for some of their products. Although OpenCL unifies high-performance programming in a single language it seems unlikely that a single OpenCL program is able to deliver the best possible performance on different acceleration platforms.

We only looked at the most time-consuming parts of iterative reconstruction methods. The implementation of a specific iterative method may introduce additional problems both concerning the efficient parallel implementation and the algorithmic building blocks. For example, there are other choices for implementing the forward-projection step than ray casting.

Finally, other reconstruction algorithms may be applied to solve the 3-D CT reconstruction task. For example, there are theoretically exact and stable methods that can better deal with truncated projections. In this regard, differentiated back-projection filtration (DBF) approaches may be worth to be considered. Helical CT reconstruction algorithms are another topic of research we have excluded from our considerations. In several helical CT scanners cylindrical detectors are installed that require a special treatment of that geometry.

Appendix A

Geometry Parameter Extraction

For mechanically unstable cone-beam CT scanners the scan geometry slightly deviates from that of an ideal scan. These deviations are often not negligible [Wies 00]. In order to achieve good image quality also for non-ideal acquisitions the imaging geometry has to be defined accurately for each acquired projection image.

The imaging geometry for the X-ray camera at position $\underline{a}(\lambda)$ can be defined by a 3×4 projection matrix for which the left hand 3×3 sub-matrix is non-singular [Hart 03]. To extract the geometrical parameters from a projection matrix $\mathbf{P}(\lambda)$ we need to decompose $\mathbf{P}(\lambda)$ into the following product

$$\mathbf{P}(\lambda) = \mathbf{K}(\lambda) \left[\ \mathbf{R}(\lambda) \quad -\mathbf{R}(\lambda)\underline{a}(\lambda) \ \right] , \tag{A.1}$$

where the calibration matrix $\mathbf{K}(\lambda)$ is of the form

$$\mathbf{K}(\lambda) = \begin{bmatrix} \frac{D}{du} & s & \check{u}_0 \\ 0 & \frac{D}{dv} & \check{v}_0 \\ 0 & 0 & 1 \end{bmatrix} . \tag{A.2}$$

The parameter s is referred to as the *skew* parameter. A non-zero value of s corresponds to a sheared detector pixel grid.

The rotation matrix

$$\mathbf{R}(\lambda) = \left[\ \underline{e}_u(\lambda) \quad \underline{e}_v(\lambda) \quad -\underline{e}_w(\lambda) \ \right]^T \tag{A.3}$$

consists of the unit vectors that define the detector coordinate system. In order to obtain $\mathbf{K}(\lambda)$, $\mathbf{R}(\lambda)$ and $\underline{a}(\lambda)$ from $\mathbf{P}(\lambda)$ we reformulate Equation (A.1) into

$$\mathbf{P}(\lambda) = \left[\ \mathbf{M}(\lambda) \quad -\mathbf{M}(\lambda)\underline{a}(\lambda) \ \right] , \tag{A.4}$$

where the matrix $\mathbf{M}(\lambda) = \mathbf{K}(\lambda)\mathbf{R}(\lambda)$ is the left hand 3×3 sub-matrix of $\mathbf{P}(\lambda)$.[1]

Finally, the source position $\underline{a}(\lambda)$ is computed according to

$$\underline{a}(\lambda) = -\mathbf{M}^{-1}\mathbf{P}(\lambda)[:,3] . \tag{A.5}$$

The inversion of matrix $\mathbf{M}(\lambda)$ can be done in a numerically stable way e.g. by using a singular value decomposition [Golu 96].

---

[1] The matrix $\mathbf{M}(\lambda)$ can be decomposed as $\mathbf{M}(\lambda) = \mathbf{K}(\lambda)\mathbf{R}(\lambda)$ where $\mathbf{M}(\lambda)$ is upper triangular and $\mathbf{R}(\lambda)$ is orthogonal. This decomposition is essentially the RQ matrix decomposition (see [Hart 03] for further details).

Appendix B

Datasets

In this thesis the computational performance has been evaluated using two clinical datasets acquired with C-arm systems.

The projection images have been preprocessed using the "RenderDib" tool from the AX department of Siemens Healthcare. The preprocessed images have been written as raw float arrays to separate files. The relevant calibration information and the description of the maximum volume of interest were available from a previous calibration. In case of the Feldkamp algorithm we further applied cosine and Parker weighting to the projection images.

In the following we briefly summarize the details of these datasets.

B.1 Dataset (a): Head

Dataset (a) consisted of 414 projection images of 1024×1024 pixels each. The convolution length for the Fourier-based filtering step was 2048 including zero padding for this dataset. In the back-projection step of the Feldkamp algorithm the isotropic voxel size was set to 0.26^3 mm^3 so that the whole volume was located inside the FOV. During the evaluations of the iterative approach the volume contained the complete FOV thus using a voxel size of 0.38^3 mm^3. The reconstructed volume shows a human head (see Figure B.1).

B.2 Dataset (b): Hip Junction

Dataset (b) consisted of 543 projection images of 1240×960 pixels each. During the evaluations of the Feldkamp algorithm the convolution length was 4096 and the isotropic voxel size 0.31^3 mm^3. For the iterative approaches the volume was configured with a voxel size of 0.46^3 mm^3. The reconstructed volume shows a phantom of a human hip (see Figure B.2).

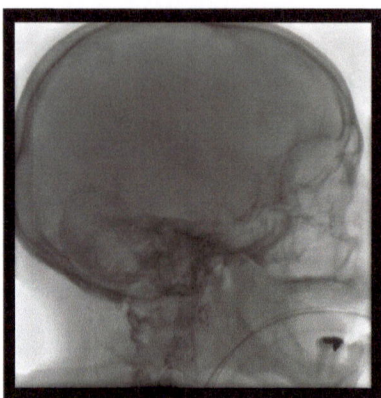

(a) Projection image.

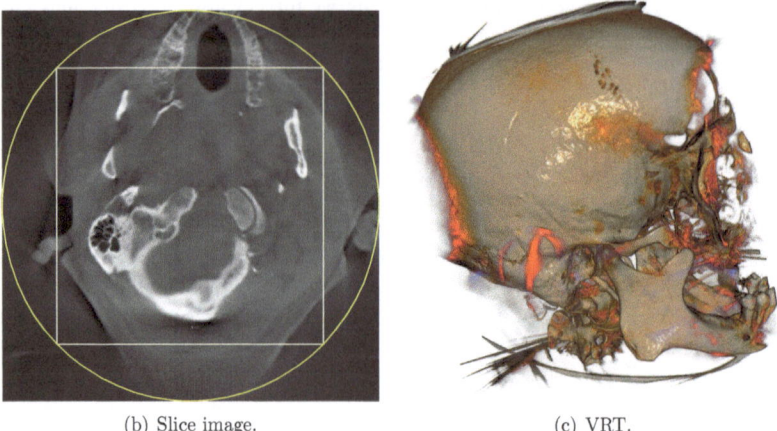

(b) Slice image.   (c) VRT.

Figure B.1: Dataset (a) – Head. A single projection image of the dataset is shown (a). The projection images of this dataset show a border of zero values around each image. During reconstruction these borders have been assumed to contain image information. In (b) a reconstructed slice image is shown. It has been scaled to its full intensity range. The yellow circle indicates the FOV, while the white square indicates the region, which has been reconstructed during the performance evaluations of the FDK method. Finally, the image in (c) has been computed by a volume rendering technique (VRT).

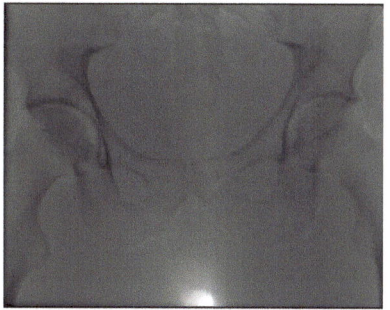

(a) Projection image.

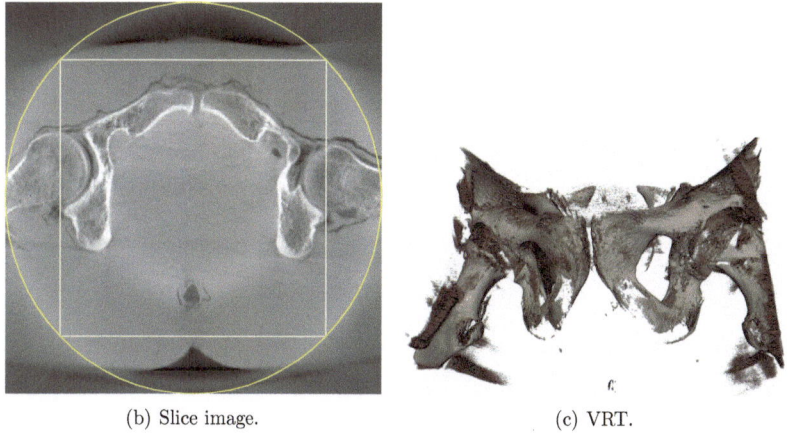

(b) Slice image. (c) VRT.

Figure B.2: Dataset (b) – Hip Junction. The images in (a) and (b) show a single projection image of the dataset and a reconstructed slice image, respectively. Both images have been scaled to their full intensity range. In (b) the yellow circle indicates the FOV, while the white square indicates the region, which has been reconstructed during the performance evaluations of the FDK method. Finally, the image in (c) has been computed by a volume rendering technique (VRT).

Appendix C

Acronyms

AMD	Advanced Micro Devices
API	Application Programming Interface
ART	Algebraic Reconstruction Technique
BIC	Bus Interface Controller
BL	Bilinear
CBEA	Cell Broadband Engine Architecture
CCS	Camera Coordinate System
CPI	Cycles Per Instruction
CPLD	Complex Programmable Logic Devices
CPU	Central Processing Unit
CT	Computed Tomography
CUDA	Compute Unified Device Architecture
CUFFT	CUDA Fast Fourier Transform
DBF	Differentiated Back-projection Filtration
DCS	Detector Coordinate System
DDR	Double Data Rate
DFT	Discrete Fourier Transform
DMA	Direct Memory Access
DRAM	Dynamic Random Access Memory
DSP	Digital Signal Processor
ECS	Extended Texture Coordinate System
EIB	Element Interconnect Bus
FDK	Reconstruction method by Feldkamp, Davis, and Kress
FFT	Fast Fourier Transform
FOV	Field-Of-View
FPGA	Field-Programmable Gate Arrays
fps	frames per second
GPU	Graphics Processing Unit
IBM	International Business Machines Corporation
IDFT	Inverse Discrete Fourier Transform
IFFT	Inverse Fast Fourier Transform
ILP	Instruction Level Parallelism
IO	Input/Output

IPP	Integrated Performance Primitives
LME	Lehrstuhl für Mustererkennung
LRR	Lehrstuhl für Rechnertechnik und Rechnerorganisation
LS	Local Store
M-line	Theoretically exact and stable reconstruction method
MFC	Memory Flow Controller
MIC	Memory Interface Controller
MLEM	Maximum Likelihood Expectation Maximization
NDT	Non-Destructive Testing
NN	Nearest Neighbor
OpenGL	Open Graphics Library
OSEM	Ordered Subset Expectation Maximization
PCI	Peripheral Component Interconnect
PCS	Pixel Coordinate System
PPE	PowerPC Processor Element
pps	projections per second
PPU	Power Processor Unit
RAM	Random Access Memory
RISC	Reduced Instruction Set Computer
RTK	Reconstruction Toolkit
SART	Simultaneous Algebraic Reconstruction Technique
SDK	Software Development Kit
SDRAM	Synchronous Dynamic Random Access Memory
SIMD	Single Instruction, Multiple Data
SIRT	Simultaneous Iterative Reconstruction Technique
SMP	Symmetric Multiprocessing
SPE	Synergistic Processor Element
SPU	Synergistic Processor Unit
SSE	Streaming SIMD Extensions
TCS	Texture Coordinate System
TLB	Translation Lookaside Buffer
TP	Thread Processor
TU	Technische Universität
UML	Unified Modeling Language
VCS	Voxel Coordinate System
VHDL	Very High Speed Integrated Circuit Description Language
VOI	Volume-Of-Interest
VPU	Vector Processing Unit
VRT	Volume Rendering Technique
WCS	World Coordinate System
WIB	Work Instruction Block

List of Figures

List of Tables

List of Algorithms

Bibliography

[Alex 01]   A. Alexandrescu. *Modern C++ Design Generic Programming and Design Patterns Applied.* Addison-Wesley, New York, 2001.

[Cell 06]   *Cell Broadband Engine Programming Handbook.* IBM, 1.0 Ed., 2006.

[Chur 07]   M. Churchill. "Hardware-Accelerated Cone-Beam Reconstruction on a Mobile C-arm". In: J. Hsieh and M. Flynn, Eds., *Proceedings of SPIE*, San Diego, March 2007.

[Cool 65]   J. Cooley and J. Tukey. "An algorithm for the machine computation of the complex Fourier series". *Mathematics of Computation*, Vol. 19, No. 50, pp. 297 – 301, April 1965.

[De M 02]   B. De Man and S. Basu. "Distance-driven projection and backprojection". In: *Nuclear Science Symposium Conference Record, 2002 IEEE*, pp. 1477 – 1480, November 2002.

[De M 04]   B. De Man and S. Basu. "Distance-driven projection and backprojection in three dimensions". *Physics in Medicine and Biology*, Vol. 49, No. 11, pp. 2463 – 2475, June 2004.

[Enge 06]   K. Engel, M. Hadwiger, J. M. Kniss, C. Rezk-Salama, and D. Weiskopf. *Real-Time Volume Graphics.* A K Peters, Ltd., 2006.

[Feld 84]   L. Feldkamp, L. Davis, and J. Kress. "Practical Cone-Beam Algorithm". *Journal of the Optical Society of America*, Vol. A1, No. 6, pp. 612–619, February 1984.

[Gali 03]   R. R. Galigekere, K. Wiesent, and D. W. Holdsworth. "Cone-Beam Reprojection Using Projection-Matrices". *IEEE Transactions on Medical Imaging*, Vol. 22, No. 10, pp. 1202–1214, October 2003.

[Gamm 94]   E. Gamma, R. Helm, R. Johnson, and J. Vlissides. *Design Patterns Elements of Reusable Object-Oriented Software.* Addison-Wesley, 1994.

[Godd 02]   I. Goddard and M. Trepanier. "High-speed cone-beam reconstruction: an embedded systems approach". In: S. Mun, Ed., *Proc. SPIE Medical Imaging 2002: Visualization, Image-Guided Procedures, and Display*, pp. 483–491, San Diego, 2002.

[Golu 96]   G. H. Golub and C. F. Van Loan. *Matrix Computations. Johns Hopkins Studies in Mathematical Sciences*, The Johns Hopkins University Press, Baltimore, 3rd Ed., 1996.

[Gonz 08]   R. C. Gonzalez and R. E. Woods. *Digital Image Processing.* Pearson Education, Inc., 3rd Ed., 2008.

[Gord 70]   R. Gordon, R. Bender, and G. Herman. "Algebraic reconstruction tech-
            niques (ART) for the three dimensional electron microscopy and X-ray
            photography". *Journal of theoretical biology*, Vol. 29, No. 3, pp. 471–481,
            August 1970.

[Gran 98]   M. Grand. *Patterns in Java, Volume 1, A Catalog of Reusable Design
            Patterns Illustrated with UML*. Wiley Computer Publishing, New York,
            1998.

[Guan 94]   H. Guan and R. Gordon. "A projection access order for speedy conver-
            gence of ART (algebraic reconstruction technique): a multilevel scheme
            for computed tomography". *Physics in Medicine and Biology*, Vol. 39,
            No. 11, pp. 2005–2022, November 1994.

[Hart 03]   R. Hartley and A. Zissermann. *Multiple View Geometry in computer
            vision*. Cambridge University Press, Cambridge, second Ed., 2003.

[Heig 07]   B. Heigl and M. Kowarschik. "High-Speed Reconstruction for C-arm com-
            puted tomography". In: *Proceedings Fully 3D Meeting and HPIR Work-
            shop*, pp. 25–28, Lindau, July 2007.

[Henn 03]   J. Hennessy and D. Patterson. *Computer Architecture: A Quantitative
            Approach*. Morgan Kaufmann, 3. Ed., 2003.

[Hill 09]   L. Hillebrand, R. Lapp, Y. Kyriakou, and W. Kalender. "Interactive
            GPU-accelerated image reconstruction in cone-beam CT". In: E. Samei
            and J. Hsieh, Eds., *Medical Imaging 2009: Physics of Medical Imaging*,
            p. 72582A, SPIE, 2009.

[Hopp 06]   S. Hoppe, F. Dennerlein, G. Lauritsch, J. Hornegger, and F. Noo. "Cone-
            beam Tomography from Short-Scan Circle-plus-Arc Data measured on a
            C-arm system". In: *IEEE Nuclear Science Symposium Conference Record*,
            pp. 2873–2877, San Diego, 2006.

[Huds 94]   H. Hudson and R. Larkin. "Accelerated image reconstruction using or-
            dered subsets of projection data". *IEEE Transactions on Medical Imaging*,
            Vol. 13, No. 4, pp. 601–609, December 1994.

[John 07]   S. G. Johnson and M. Frigo. "A modified split-radix FFT with fewer
            arithmetic operations". *IEEE Transactions on Signal Processing*, Vol. 55,
            No. 1, pp. 111–119, January 2007.

[Jose 83]   P. Joseph. "An improved algorithm for reprojecting rays through pixel
            images". *IEEE Transactions on Medical Imaging*, Vol. 1, No. 3, pp. 192–
            196, 1983.

[Kach 06]   M. Kachelrieß, M. Knaup, and O. Bockenbach. "Hyperfast Perspective
            Cone-Beam Backprojection". In: *IEEE Nuclear Science Symposium and
            Medical Imaging Conference*, San Diego, 2006. M01-7.

[Kach 07]   M. Kachelrieß, M. Knaup, and O. Bockenbach. "Hyperfast parallel-beam
            and cone-beam backprojection using the Cell general purpose hardware".
            Medical Physics, Vol. 34, No. 4, pp. 1474–1486, March 2007.

[Kacz 37]   S. Kaczmarz. "Angenäherte Auflösung von Systemen linearer Gleichun-
            gen". *Bulletin International de l'Academie Polonaise des Sciences et des
            Lettres*, Vol. 6-8A, pp. 335–357, 1937.

[Kak 01]   A. Kak and M. Slaney. *Principles of Computerized Tomographic Imaging.* SIAM, 2001.

[Kats 03]   A. Katsevich. "A general Scheme for constructing Inversion Algorithms for Cone Beam CT". *International Journal of Mathematics and Mathematical Sciences,* Vol. 2003, No. 21, pp. 1305–1321, April 2003.

[Kats 04]   A. Katsevich. "Image Reconstruction for the Circle and Line Trajectory". *Physics in Medicine and Biology,* Vol. 49, No. 22, pp. 5059–5072, October 2004.

[Kats 05]   A. Katsevich. "Image Reconstruction for the Circle-and-Arc Trajectory". *Physics in Medicine and Biology,* Vol. 50, No. 10, pp. 2249–2265, April 2005.

[Keck 09a] B. Keck, H. Hofmann, H. Scherl, M. Kowarschik, and J. Hornegger. "GPU-accelerated SART reconstruction using the CUDA programming environment". In: E. Samei and J. Hsieh, Eds., *Medical Imaging 2009: Physics of Medical Imaging,* p. 72582B, February 2009.

[Keck 09b] B. Keck, H. Hofmann, H. Scherl, M. Kowarschik, and J. Hornegger. "High Resolution Iterative CT Reconstruction using Graphics Hardware". In: B. Yu, Ed., *2009 IEEE Nuclear Science Symposium Conference Record,* pp. 4035–4040, 2009.

[Laur 98]   C. Laurent, F. Peyrin, J. M. Chassery, and M. Amiel. "Parallel image reconstruction on MIMD computers for three-dimensional cone-beam tomography". *Parallel Computing,* Vol. 24, No. 9-10, pp. 1461–1479, 1998.

[Lian 10]   W. Liang, H. Zhang, and G. Hu. "Optimized Implementation of the FDK Algorithm on One Digital Signal Processor". *Tsinghua Science and Technology,* Vol. 15, No. 1, pp. 108 – 113, 2010.

[Matt 05]   T. G. Mattson, B. A. Sanders, and B. L. Massingill. *Patterns for parallel programming.* Addison-Wesley, Boston, 2005.

[Meye 08]   U. Meyer-Bäse. *Digital Signal Processing with Field Programmable Gate Arrays (Signals and Communication Technology).* Springer, Berlin, Heidelberg, New York, 2nd Ed., 2008.

[Muel 07]   K. Mueller, F. Xu, and N. Neophytou. "Why do Commodity Graphics Hardware Boards (GPUs) work so well for acceleration of Computed Tomography?". In: *SPIE Electronic Imaging Conference,* San Diego, 2007. (Keynote, Computational Imaging V).

[Muel 98]   K. Mueller. *Fast and Accurate Three-Dimensional Reconstruction from Cone-Beam Projection Data using Algebraic Methods.* PhD thesis, School of The Ohio State University, 1998.

[Neri 07]   R. A. Neri-Calderón, S. Alcaraz-Corona, and R. M. Rodríguez-Dagnino. "Cache-optimized implementation of the filtered backprojection algorithm on a digital signal processor". *Journal of Electronic Imaging,* Vol. 16, No. 4, p. 043010, 2007.

[Noo 03]   F. Noo and D. Heuscher. "Exact helical reconstruction using native cone-beam geometries". *Physics in Medicine and Biology,* Vol. 48, No. 23, pp. 3787–3818, 2003.

[Noo 09]   F. Noo. "Analytical image reconstruction methods II: 3D cone-beam tomography". Short Course at the 10th International Meeting on Fully Three-Dimensional Image Reconstruction in Radiology and Nuclear Medicine, September 2009.

[NVID 09]   *NVIDIA CUDA Programming Guide - Version 2.3.1.* NVIDIA Corporation, 2701 San Tomas Expressway, Santa Clara, CA 95050, USA, 2009.

[Oh 06]   H.-J. Oh, S. Mueller, C. Jacobi, K. Tran, S. Cottier, B. Michael, H. Nishikawa, Y. Totsuka, T. Namatame, N. Yano, T. Machida, and S. Dhong. "A fully pipelined single-precision floating-point unit in the synergistic processor element of a CELL processor". *IEEE Journal of Solid-State Circuits*, Vol. 41, No. 4, pp. 759–771, 2006.

[Pack 05]   J. Pack and F. Noo. "Cone-beam reconstruction using 1D filtering along the projection of M-lines". *Inverse Problems*, Vol. 21, No. 3, pp. 1105–1120, 2005.

[Park 82]   D. L. Parker. "Optimal short scan convolution reconstruction for fan beam CT". *Medical Physics*, Vol. 9, No. 2, pp. 254–257, March 1982.

[Pham 05]   D. Pham, S. Asano, M. Bolliger, M. Day, H. Hofstee, C. Johns, J. Kahle, A. Kameyama, J. Keaty, Y. Masubuchi, M. Riley, D. Shippy, D. Stasiak, M. Suzuoki, M. Wang, J. Warnock, S. Weitzel, D. Wendel, T. Yamazaki, and K. Yazawa. "The design and implementation of a first-generation CELL processor". In: *IEEE Solid-State Circuits Conference*, pp. 184–185, San Francisco, 2005.

[Posn 96]   E. J. Posnak, R. G. Lavender, and H. M. Vin. "Adaptive pipeline: an object structural pattern for adaptive applications". In: *The 3rd Pattern Languages of Programming conference*, Monticello, Illinois, September 1996.

[Reim 96]   D. Reimann, V. Chaudhary, M. Flynn, and I. Sethi. "(C) Parallel Implementation of Cone Beam Tomography". In: *ICPP '96: Proceedings of the 1996 International Conference on Parallel Processing*, p. 0170, IEEE Computer Society, Los Alamitos, CA, USA, 1996.

[Ridd 06]   C. Riddell and Y. Trousset. "Rectification for Cone-Beam Projection and Backprojection". *IEEE Transactions on Medical Imaging*, Vol. 25, No. 7, pp. 950–962, 2006.

[Sche 05]   H. Scherl, M. Kowarschik, and J. Hornegger. "Bit-Accurate Simulation of Convolution-Based Filtering on Reconfigurable Hardware". In: F. Hülsemann, M. Kowarschik, and U. Rüde, Eds., *Frontiers in Simulation*, pp. 662–667, Erlangen, 2005.

[Sche 07a] H. Scherl, S. Hoppe, F. Dennerlein, G. Lauritsch, W. Eckert, M. Kowarschik, and J. Hornegger. "On-the-fly reconstruction in exact cone-beam CT using the Cell Broadband Engine Architecture". In: *Proceedings Fully 3D Meeting and HPIR Workshop*, pp. 29–32, Lindau, July 2007.

[Sche 07b] H. Scherl, B. Keck, M. Kowarschik, and J. Hornegger. "Fast GPU-Based CT Reconstruction using the Common Unified Device Architecture (CUDA)". In: E. C. Frey, Ed., *Nuclear Science Symposium, Medical Imaging Conference 2007*, pp. 4464–4466, 2007.

[Sche 07c] H. Scherl, M. Koerner, H. Hofmann, W. Eckert, M. Kowarschik, and J. Hornegger. "Implementation of the FDK Algorithm for Cone-Beam CT on the Cell Broadband Engine Architecture". In: J. Hsieh and M. Flynn, Eds., *Medical Imaging 2007: Physics of Medical Imaging*, p. 651058, February 2007.

[Sche 08] H. Scherl, S. Hoppe, M. Kowarschik, and J. Hornegger. "Design and implementation of the software architecture for a 3-D reconstruction system in medical imaging". In: W. Schäfer, M. B. Dwyer, and V. Gruhn, Eds., *ICSE '08: Proceedings of the 30th international conference on Software engineering*, pp. 661–668, New York, NY, USA, 2008.

[Scho 01] H. Schomberg. "Complete Source Trajectories for C-Arm Systems and a Method for Coping with Truncated Cone-Beam Projections". In: *Sixth International Meeting on Fully Three-Dimensional Image Reconstruction in Radiology and Nuclear Medicine*, pp. 221–224, Pacific Grove, CA, USA, October 30 - November 2 2001.

[Seil 08] L. Seiler, D. Carmean, E. Sprangle, T. Forsyth, M. Abrash, P. Dubey, S. Junkins, A. Lake, J. Sugerman, R. Cavin, R. Espasa, E. Grochowski, T. Juan, and P. Hanrahan. "Larrabee: A Many-Core x86 Architecture for Visual Computing". In: *SIGGRAPH '08: ACM SIGGRAPH 2008 papers*, pp. 1–15, ACM, Los Angeles, Aug. 2008.

[Shep 82] L. Shepp and Y. Vardi. "Maximum likelihood reconstruction for emission tomography". *IEEE Transactions on Medical Imaging*, Vol. 1, No. 2, pp. 113–122, October 1982.

[Sidd 85] R. L. Siddon. "Fast calculation of the exact radiological path for a three-dimensional CT array". *Medical Physics*, Vol. 12, No. 2, pp. 252–255, March/April 1985.

[Silv 00] M. D. Silver. "A method for including redundant data in computed tomography". *Medical Physics*, Vol. 27, No. 4, pp. 773–774, April 2000.

[Syne 05] *Synergistic Processing Unit Instruction Set Architecture*. IBM, 1.0 Ed., 2005.

[Trep 02] M. Trepanier and I. Goddard. "Adjunct processors in embedded medical imaging systems". In: S. Mun, Ed., *Proc. SPIE Medical Imaging 2002: Visualization, Image-Guided Procedures, and Display*, pp. 416–424, 2002.

[Turb 01] H. Turbell. *Cone-Beam Reconstruction Using Filtered Backprojection*. PhD thesis, Linköping University, Sweden, SE-581 83 Linköping, Sweden, February 2001. Dissertation No. 672, ISBN 91-7219-919-9.

[Tuy 83] H. Tuy. "An inversion formula for cone-beam reconstruction". *SIAM J. Appl. Math.*, Vol. 43, No. 3, pp. 546–552, 1983.

[Verm 95] A. Vermeulen, G. Beged-Dov, and P. Thompson. "The pipeline design pattern". In: *OOPSLA'95 Workshop on Design Patterns for Concurrent, Parallel and Distributed Object-Oriented Systems*, October 1995.

[Wein 08] A. Weinlich, B. Keck, H. Scherl, M. Kowarschik, and J. Hornegger. "Comparison of High-Speed Ray Casting on GPU using CUDA and OpenGL". In: R. Buchty and J.-P. Weiß, Eds., *Proceedings of the First International Workshop on New Frontiers in High-performance and Hardware-aware Computing (HipHaC'08)*, pp. 25–30, Karlsruhe, 2008.

[Welc 69]   P. Welch. "A Fixed–Point Fast Fourier Transform Error Analysis". *IEEE Transactions on Audio and Electroacoustics*, Vol. 17, No. 2, 1969.

[Wies 00]   K. Wiesent, K. Barth, N. Navab, P. Durlak, T. Brunner, O. Schuetz, and W. Seissler. "Enhanced 3-D-reconstruction algorithm for C-arm systems suitable for interventional procedures". *IEEE Transactions on Medical Imaging*, Vol. 19, No. 5, pp. 391–403, 2000.

[Xu 06]   F. Xu and K. Mueller. "A comparative study of popular interpolation and integration methods for use in computed tomography". In: *Proceedings of the 2006 IEEE International Symposium on Biomedical Imaging: From Nano to Macro, Arlington, VA, USA, 6-9 April 2006*, pp. 1252–1255, IEEE, 2006.

[Xu 07]   F. Xu and K. Mueller. "Real-time 3D computed tomographic reconstruction using commodity graphics hardware". *Physics in Medicine and Biology*, Vol. 52, pp. 3405–3419, July 2007.

[Yan 08]   G. Yan, S. Zhu, Y. Dai, and C. Qin. "Fast cone-beam CT image reconstruction using GPU hardware". *Journal of X-Ray Science and Technology*, Vol. 16, pp. 225–234, July 2008.

[Yu 01]   R. Yu, R. Ning, and B. Chen. "High-speed cone-beam reconstruction on PC". In: M. Sonka and K. Hanson, Eds., *Proc. SPIE Medical Imaging 2001: Image Processing*, pp. 964–973, San Diego, 2001.

[Zbij 03]   F. Zbijewski, W. Beekman. "FBP initialization for transition artifacts reduction in statistical X-ray CT reconstruction". In: *Nuclear Science Symposium Conference Record, 2003 IEEE*, pp. 2970–2972, October 2003.

[Zell 05]   M. Zellerhoff, B. Scholz, E.-P. Rührnschopf, and T. Brunner. "Low contrast 3-D-reconstruction from C-arm data". In: M. J. Flynn, Ed., *Proceedings of SPIE*, pp. 646–655, April 2005.

[Zeng 00]   G. L. Zeng and G. T. Gullberg. "Unmatched Projector/Backprojector Pairs in an Iterative Reconstruction Algorithm". *IEEE Transactions on Medical Imaging*, Vol. 19, No. 5, pp. 548–555, May 2000.

[Zhan 06]   Y. Zhang, H.-P. Chan, B. Sahiner, J. Wei, M. M. Goodsitt, L. M. Hadjiiski, J. Ge, and C. Zhou. "A comparative study of limited-angle cone-beam reconstruction methods for breast tomosynthesis". *Medical Physics*, Vol. 33, No. 10, pp. 3781–3795, 2006.